Chinese System of Natural Cures

Henry C. Lu, Ph.D.

STERLING PUBLISHING CO., INC.
NEW YORK

About the Author   Dr. Henry C. Lu received his Ph.D. from the University of Alberta, Edmonton, Canada. He taught at the University of Alberta and the University of Calgary between 1968 and 1971, and he has practised Chinese medicine since 1972. Dr. Lu now teaches Chinese medicine by correspondence. His students live in many countries, including the United States, Canada, England, Australia, Sweden, Italy, Germany, France, New Zealand, Switzerland, Mexico, and Japan.

The author is best known for his translation of *The Yellow Emperor's Classics of Internal Medicine* from Chinese into English and for the International College of Traditional Chinese Medicine he established in Vancouver and Victoria, British Columbia, Canada, for the instruction of traditional Chinese medicine.

Other Sterling books by the author are *Chinese System of Food Cures, Chinese Foods for Longevity,* and *Chinese Herbal Cures.*

Dr. Lu has practised traditional Chinese medicine for more than 20 years. He invented herbal formulas in powdered and tablet form for his patients at his Vancouver clinic, and he teaches his students how to make these powdered and tablet formulas.

Dr. Lu lives and operates a clinic in Vancouver, British Columbia. Correspondence to Dr. Lu should be addressed to Dr. Henry C. Lu, P.O. Box 337, Blaine, WA, U.S.A. 98230.

Library of Congress Cataloging-in-Publication Data

Lu, Henry C.
    Chinese system of natural cures / Henry C. Lu.
      p.   cm.
    Includes index.
    ISBN 0-8069-0616-2
    1. Medicine, Chinese.   I. Title.
    R601.L875   1994
    610'.951—dc20   94-13706
                                   CIP

Edited by Laurel Ornitz

10 9 8 7 6 5 4 3 2

Published by Sterling Publishing Company, Inc.
387 Park Avenue South, New York, N.Y. 10016
© 1994 by Henry C. Lu
Distributed in Canada by Sterling Publishing
% Canadian Manda Group, P.O. Box 920, Station U
Toronto, Ontario, Canada M8Z 5P9
Distributed in Great Britain and Europe by Cassell PLC
Villiers House, 41/47 Strand, London WC2N 5JE, England
Distributed in Australia by Capricorn Link (Australia) Pty Ltd.
P.O. Box 6651, Baulkham Hills, Business Centre, NSW 2153, Australia
Manufactured in United States of America
All rights reserved

Sterling ISBN 0-8069-0616-2

CONTENTS

INTRODUCTION

T o cure a disease, in its truest sense, means to get rid of the disease so that it won't come back any more. You may have a headache and take some medication to cure it, and, after a while, the headache is gone for good. This means that your headache is cured. However, you may have a headache and take some medication to cure it, but the medication relieves your headache for only a few hours, and you need to take the medication on a regular basis in order to be free from the headache. This means that your headache is merely relieved, not cured.

If one has hypertension and has to take medication every day as long as one lives just to keep one's blood pressure down, then the medication is merely relieving the hypertension, not curing it. It is a fact that a patient with hypertension needs to take medication as long as he or she lives, not to cure the hypertension, but just to keep his or her blood pressure down; likewise, a diabetic has to take insulin as long as he or she lives, not to cure the diabetes, but just to keep his or her blood sugar or urine sugar down.

These examples reflect the Western approach to the treatment of diseases, but the Chinese approach is different, as it is always aimed at curing the diseases, not simply relieving the symptoms. How does Chinese medicine achieve this aim? It does so through an understanding of symptoms by way of syndromes.

A syndrome is a group of symptoms collectively involved in a particular disease. Take hypertension, for example. In Western medicine, hypertension, or high blood pressure, is understood as an isolated symptom and treated as such. For this reason, every patient with hypertension is treated basically the same way with the same drugs. In other words, to a typical Western doctor, hypertension is hypertension, whether it attacks Mr. Smith or Ms. Anderson. Any drug considered effective for one patient with hypertension is considered effective for all patients with hypertension. This is not the case in Chinese medicine, in which a given herb or food may be effective in treating Mr. Smith's hypertension but not Ms. Anderson's.

Some patients with hypertension may have headache or dizziness; others may have ringing in the ears or blurred vision; still others may have perspiration or fatigue. From the point of view of Chinese medicine, *all* the symptoms a patient displays should be taken into account, not just hypertension, in order to develop an adequate form of treatment.

The Chinese have coined different terminologies to name a wide variety of syndromes. These include liver yang upsurging, yin deficiency of the kidneys, lungs-dampness, and no communication between the heart and the kidneys. No doubt, these terms are new to most Westerners and may seem strange. However,

5

each discipline needs terminologies; you may gradually find the Chinese terms extremely useful in understanding diseases.

Since each disorder will be understood by means of the syndromes involved in it, and since we will be treating the predominant syndrome in dealing with a disorder, you need to be able to differentiate syndromes for the disorders.

Here is how to do it, using hypertension (pages 107–108) as an example. Hypertension may arise from the following three syndromes: 1. liver-fire, 2. liver and kidneys yin deficiency, and 3. both yin and yang are deficient. As you can see below, each syndrome is defined by a variety of symptoms, followed by a number within brackets. Assuming that you are a patient with hypertension, underline all the symptoms you have repeatedly under each syndrome; then add up all the numbers of the symptoms you have underlined under each syndrome to arrive at your score for each one. For your convenience, **following each syndrome** name there is an **empty set of brackets**, in which you can **pencil in the score**.

Let's suppose you are experiencing the following symptoms: blood pressure rises easily with anger or stress, severe headache, insomnia, hot temper, dry mouth, many dreams, red eyes, and lumbago. You should **underline these symptoms**, and **record your total score in the brackets** after the syndrome name.

1. Liver-fire syndrome (12)

The symptoms: blood pressure rises readily with anger or stress (4), severe headache (2), vertigo (2), red face (2), red eyes (2), hot temper (2), bitter taste in the mouth (2), dry mouth (2), discharge of yellowish and scant urine (2)

2. Liver and kidneys yin deficiency with liver yang upsurging syndrome (7)

The symptoms: blood pressure rises readily with fatigue and stress (3), vertigo (2), ringing in the ears (2), insomnia (2), many dreams (2), hot temper (1), discharge of reddish and scant urine (2), lumbago (2), pain in the legs (1), seminal emission (2), numbness of the four limbs (1)

3. Both yin and yang are deficient with deficient yang moving upward syndrome (3)

The symptoms: light headache (1), vertigo (1), blurred vision (1), ringing in the ears (2), slightly red face (1), dry mouth (1), perspiration (1), insomnia (1), many dreams (1), cold limbs (2), lumbago (1), weak legs (1), frequent urination at night (2), twitching of muscles (2), heavy breathing upon walking (2)

Since you scored 12 for the first syndrome, 7 for the second syndrome, and 3 for the third syndrome, it is clear that your hypertension falls within the first syndrome (liver-fire), so you should treat your ailments accordingly.

As to the treatment, there is a difference between treatment with herbs and foods. Herbs are used to *correct* the weakness and imbalance in the body, and the internal organs in particular, so that the body and internal organs will be strong and in balance, whereas foods are used to *maintain* the strength and balance. This is why we don't eat herbs every day or for a very long period of time, but we eat foods every day. To take medication every day and as long as one lives is to mix up drugs with foods, but a similar mix-up does not exist in Chinese medicine. Patients often ask me whether they should take herbs forever or how long they should take them. My answer is always that as soon as they have achieved the strength and balance of their body through herbs, they should stop taking them and instead eat appropriate foods to maintain this strength and balance.

When you go through the symptoms under each heading, you will come across symptoms followed by an asterisk (*) or in italics. The symptoms with an asterisk are the most crucial symptoms in making a diagnosis; those in italics are the next most crucial. The following symptoms are taken from under the heading of Hypotension (pages 108–110):

Hypotension

1. Heart yang deficiency syndrome (　)

Symptoms:
Cold sensations (1)
Fatigue (1)
Getting scared easily with rapid heartbeats (1)
Female patient (3)*
Hands and feet extremely cold (1)
Over sixty years old (3)*
Pain in the chest (2)
Pain in the heart (2)
Palpitations with insecure feeling (1)
Perspiring heavily (1)
Systolic pressure below 90 mm of mercury (3)*
Unconsciousness (1)

Two symptoms are followed by an asterisk—namely, female patient and over sixty years old. Each of them is given 3 points to indicate their importance in making the diagnosis. Three symptoms are in italics—pain in the chest, pain in the heart, and palpitations with insecure feeling—and each is given 2 points, indicating their relative importance.

1
THE SYSTEM
OF TRADITIONAL
CHINESE MEDICINE

ALTHOUGH TRADITIONAL Chinese medicine is as old as Chinese history itself, if it is new to you, you will likely have many questions about this type of medicine and what it can offer you for your good health. This brief overview of its philosophy and components will help you understand it quickly.

Traditional Chinese medicine includes four distinct methods of treatment: herbology, acupuncture, manipulative therapy, and food cures. In addition, it encompasses the remedial exercises *qi-gong,* and *tai-ji.*

Traditional Chinese medicine goes back over 3,000 years. It was not developed by any particular individual; rather, it grew out of the necessity of maintaining good health among the Chinese people. The ancient Chinese, like all of us, had to struggle against diseases in order to stay in good health. In the process, they came to see the benefits of consuming herbs (known as Chinese herbology today), inserting needles in the body (known as Chinese acupuncture today), eating the right foods (known as Chinese food cures today), massaging the body (known as Chinese manipulative therapy today), and exercising the body (known as *qi-gong* and *tai-ji*).

Today, traditional Chinese medicine is practised in China side by side with modern Western medicine. There are as many hospitals of traditional Chinese medicine as modern hospitals of Western medicine. From the Chinese point of view, traditional Chinese medicine is on an equal footing with Western medicine; in fact, many Chinese value traditional Chinese medicine over Western medicine.

You may ask why we need traditional Chinese medicine when modern, scientific medicine is available to all of us. The reason is that many diseases and ailments that cannot be cured by Western medicine can be treated by traditional Chinese medicine successfully. It is a fact that many patients experience instant relief of pain when treated with Chinese acupuncture, which cannot be achieved by Western medicine. In addition, traditional Chinese medicine has proven superior to Western medicine in the treatment of skin, liver, and kidneys diseases, as well as many other diseases.

When you go to see a doctor of traditional Chinese medicine, the doctor will observe your complexion and look at your tongue, take your pulse, and ask you many questions about your symptoms, your eating habits, and your food preferences. Then the doctor will come up with a diagnosis of what is wrong with your body and tell you whether you need acupuncture or herbs and what foods are good for you.

In China, virtually all kinds of disorders are treated by traditional Chinese medicine. Some disorders may be more effectively treated by acupuncture, others by herbs; still others may be best treated by food cures. In general, pain and muscular symptoms are more effectively treated by acupuncture, skin diseases and diseases of internal organs by herbs. However, it is necessary for a doctor of traditional Chinese medicine to make a diagnosis before deciding what type of treatment would be most effective for a particular patient. When a Western doctor tells a patient that there is no cure for a certain disease, it does not necessarily mean that the disease in question cannot be cured by treatments in traditional Chinese medicine either; it only means that there is no cure for the disease by methods of Western medicine.

There are a number of basic differences between the two distinct types of medicine. First of all, Western medicine focuses more on the treatment of symptoms, whereas traditional Chinese medicine focuses more on causes. Western medicine is more useful for first aid and surgery, while traditional Chinese medicine is more useful in treating skin and internal diseases, and chronic cases in particular. Many remedies in Western medicine are based upon the results of experiments with animals which may not be effective with the human body. But remedies in traditional Chinese medicine are based upon successful experiences in clinical practice, which are more reliable. Most Western chemical drugs are strong and tend to produce serious side effects. On the other hand, Chinese herbs, acupuncture, and food cures are less drastic, can be longer-lasting in effects, and, when used the right way, generally do not produce side effects.

Although traditional Chinese medicine and Western medicine operate very differently, it is wise to consult a Western medical doctor in order to get a diagnosis, which may be of some use to a doctor of traditional Chinese medicine, and to get the best possible medical care available in modern society.

Traditional Chinese medicine is based, first and foremost, on a classic published in the third century B.C., entitled *Nei-Jing,* or *The Yellow Emperor's Classics of Internal Medicine.* Western medical books often become obsolete in the course of time (most likely within a few years), but many books on traditional Chinese medicine written by Chinese physicians in the past have become timeless classics. The following passage from the above-mentioned celebrated classic may shed some light on the nature of Chinese medicine: "The disease of the five viscera may be compared to a sharp needle in the skin, a stained chair, a knot, or a deposit of mud and sand in a river. One can still remove a needle from the skin, no matter how long ago it was used to prick the body. One can still wash off a stain, no matter how long it has been on the chair. One can still untie a knot, no matter how long ago it was tied. One can still remove a deposit of mud and sand in a river, no matter how long it has been there. Some people assume that a disease cannot be cured, simply because it has a long history, but the truth of the matter is that an outstanding physician can cure a disease for the same reason that one can pull a needle from the skin, wash off a stain from the chair, untie a knot, or clear the blockage from a river. A chronic disease with a very long history can still be cured, and those who think otherwise have not really mastered the art of acupuncture."

PHILOSOPHY

Yin and Yang

Yin and yang are the two most fundamental concepts in Chinese medical philosophy. Rooted in ancient Chinese philosophy, these two opposing concepts are used to account for changes in the universe in a comprehensive manner.

In anatomy, the human body is divided into yin and yang as follows: The internal region is yin, while the external region is yang; the five viscera are yin, while the six bowels are yang; and the tendons and bones are yin, while the skin is yang. In physiology, yin stands for storage of energy, while yang stands for human activities, because yin stays within like a traditional housewife while yang stays in the superficial region to guard against foreign invasion.

In pathology, yin and yang are used to describe two basic patterns of change. When yin wins a victory, yang will be diseased; when yang wins a victory, yin will be diseased. When yang wins a victory, there will be fever; when yin wins a victory, there will be chill. When yang is in deficiency, it will cause chill sensations in the superficial region; when yin is in deficiency, there will be internal heat. In diagnosis, yin and yang symptoms are used to describe the nature of a disease. According to *The Yellow Emperor's Classics of Internal Medicine,* "A good physician who has mastered the technique of diagnosis will examine the patient's color and take his pulse, and he will classify all symptoms into yin and yang as the first step in making a diagnosis."

In terms of treatment, striking a balance between yin and yang is the most fundamental principle of clinical practice. Among the treatments based on this principle are sedating the excess and toning up the deficiency. *The Yellow Emperor's Classics of Internal Medicine* states, "A hot disease should be treated by cold herbs; a cold disease should be treated by hot herbs. . . . Yin should be treated in a yang disease; yang should be treated in a yin disease."

The Five Elements

The five elements are a concept in ancient Chinese philosophy referring to the nature of materials as well as their interrelationships. The concept was later introduced into Chinese medical philosophy for clinical applications. The five elements refer to wood, fire, earth, metal, and water. In Chinese medical philosophy, the five-elements theory consists of four laws governing the relationships among the five materials.

According to this theory, the five viscera are viewed as the key organs and the four laws are applied to them. The four laws are the laws of production, control, attack, and resisting control. The correspondence between the five elements and the five viscera is as follows: Wood corresponds to the liver, tendons, and eyes. Fire corresponds to the heart, blood vessels, and tongue. Earth corresponds to the spleen, flesh, and mouth. Metal corresponds to the lungs, skin, hair, and nose. And water corresponds to the kidneys, bones, and ears.

The laws of production and control are used to illustrate the interrelationships among the viscera. For instance, the liver controls the spleen (which is called wood controlling earth), the spleen produces the lungs (which is called earth producing metal), and the lungs control the liver (which is called metal controlling wood). Thus, there are patterns of relationship among the five viscera according to the laws.

The laws of attack and resisting control are used to describe pathological changes as well as methods of treatment. For example, since liver disease will affect the spleen, it is called wood attacking earth and should be treated by inhibiting wood and supporting earth. And in treating lungs energy deficiency syndrome, it is necessary to strengthen the spleen and tone up the lungs, which is called developing earth in order to produce metal.

The five-elements theory is based upon clinical experiences and very useful in clinical practice. The four laws of the theory can be summarized as follows:

The first law, the law of production, states that one organ can produce another organ, which indicates a mother-child relationship between the two organs. The mother organ is capable of assisting the child organ in its capacity for growth and nourishment. According to this law, wood produces fire, fire produces earth, earth produces metal, metal produces water, and water produces wood.

The law of control states that one organ can control another organ. According to this law, wood controls earth, earth controls water, water controls fire, fire controls metal, and metal controls wood.

The law of attack states that one organ can attack another organ, which means that one organ may abuse its power of control and attack another organ. Thus, an abuse of the second law will lead to the application of this third law. As an example, when the energy of wood is in excess and, at the same time, metal fails to control wood properly, wood will manage to attack earth, which may cause liver-wood in excess with spleen-earth in deficiency. The law of attack falls within the context of pathology.

The fourth law, the law of resisting control, which can also be called the law of rebellion, states that one organ may resist control by another organ, which means that the employee may resist control by the boss, so to speak. This law is a reversal of the law of control, and, thus, it falls within the context of abnormal relationships among the internal organs. As an example, under normal circumstances, metal should control wood; but if the energy of metal is in short supply, or if the energy of wood is in excess, wood may resist control by metal, which gives rise to lungs-metal in deficiency with liver-wood in excess.

Energy, Blood, and Body Fluids

Energy   Energy is the motor of all human activities; all human activities are a function of energy. When energy is disordered, it can cause various types of organ disorders; conversely, organ disorders can cause energy disorders. The disorders of energy are generally divided into two categories: deficiency and excess. Deficiency means shortage, with symptoms of low functioning and decline; excess means too much, with symptoms of congestion and blockage.

With an energy deficiency, there is a functional decline of the internal organs and a low resistance of the organism against the attack of diseases. It can be seen in chronic diseases, aging, or during the recuperating stage of acute diseases. The general symptoms of energy deficiency include white or pale complexion, fatigue, weakness, poor spirits, shortness of breath, too tired to talk, low and feeble voice, excessive perspiration, tongue in light color, and weak pulse. In order to treat it, it is necessary to tone up the energy.

An excess of energy manifests itself in energy sluggishness or stagnation. Energy should travel throughout the body without difficulty. However, various factors, including emotional stress, irregular eating, attack of external energies, and external injuries, can impact energy circulation negatively and cause energy sluggishness in the chest. They can also cause swelling of the stomach and abdomen with pain if they involve the stomach and intestine, with wandering pain occurring most frequently and swelling more severe than pain. Other symptoms include intestinal rumbling, pain getting better on belching, and pain and swelling of breasts in women. In order to treat it, it is necessary to promote the flow of energy and break up energy congestion.

Another type of energy disorder is called energy upsurging, or energy rebellion, which may be seen in cough and asthma due to lungs energy upsurging and in nausea and vomiting as a result of stomach energy upsurging.

Blood Blood is a product of water and grains undergoing energy transformation, and it is closely related to the heart, spleen, and kidneys. There are three basic types of blood disorders: blood deficiency, blood coagulation, and "hot blood."

Blood deficiency means a shortage of blood due to loss of blood or insufficient production of blood. Blood deficiency can be seen in anaemia, chronic waste disease, neurosis, parasites, and irregular menstruation, with the following symptoms: pale complexion, light color of nails, light color of tongue, and fine pulse (there may be an empty pulse after massive bleeding). In order to treat it, it is necessary to tone up the blood or strengthen the energy and tone up the blood at the same time.

Blood coagulation, or blood stasis, can be seen in coronary disease, menstrual pain, suppression of menses, extra-uterine pregnancy, external injuries, and carbuncles, with such symptoms as acute pain in the affected region, mostly prickling pain in a fixed region, and pain getting worse on pressure or local swelling with lumps, pain in the lower abdomen before menstruation, scant menstrual flow in purple-black color and in lumps, and dark purple color of tongue with ecchymosis on the tongue. In order to treat it, it is necessary to activate the blood and transform coagulations.

"Hot blood" is mostly seen in "hot" diseases of external causes, such as measles, scarlet fever, and encephalomyelitis; sometimes it can also be seen in such diseases as allergic purpura, aplastic anemia, and leukemia, as well as various diseases of bleeding. The following symptoms may be present: red swelling, bleeding, skin eruptions, premature menstruation, excessive menstrual flow in fresh-red color, mental depression, thirst, reddish urine, and constipation or fever, red tongue with a yellowish coating, and rapid pulse. In order to treat hot blood, it is necessary to cool the blood, clear up heat, and counteract toxic effects.

Body Fluids Body fluids refer to the water in the body under normal circumstances. The functions of body fluids are to water and lubricate internal organs, muscles, skin, hair, membranes, and cavities; lubricate the joints; and moisten and nourish the brain, marrow, and bones.

Body fluids can be divided into clear fluids and turbid fluids. Clear fluids are spread in the muscles and membranes to moisten the muscles, skin, and hair, as well as the cavities of the senses, namely, the eyes, ears, mouth, and nose. Perspiration and urine are products of clear fluids. Turbid fluids are spread in the internal organs to nourish such organs as the brain, marrow, and bones and to lubricate the joints, but, at the same time, they also have the function of nourishing the muscles.

The production, distribution, and excretion of body fluids go through a relatively complicated process in close relationship with the lungs, spleen, kidneys, stomach, small intestine, large intestine, and bladder. *The Yellow Emperor's Classics of Internal Medicine* states: "After food enters the stomach, its pure energy is transmitted upward to the spleen; the spleen, in turn, spreads the pure energy to flow upward to the lungs; the lungs reopen and regulate the passage of waterways in order to transmit the energy of water to the bladder below; the pure energy of water then spreads in four directions and travels to irrigate the meridians of the five viscera." This means that the source of water comes from the stomach, which transmits the pure energy to the spleen; through the transporting and transforming functions of the spleen, the fluids from the stomach are sent to the lungs, which spread the fluids to various internal organs.

When foods pass through the small intestine and the large intestine, body fluids will be absorbed through the function of the small intestine in separating the clear fluids from the turbid and the function of the large intestine in transporting and transforming waste matter. This accounts for the assertions in the classic that "the small intestine takes charge of clear body fluids" and "the large intestine takes charge of turbid body fluids." These assertions point to the connection between body fluids and the small and large intestines.

In short, the production, absorption, and transportation of body fluids are inseparable from the receiving function of the stomach and the transporting and transforming functions of the spleen. The distribution of body fluids throughout the whole body to moisten the skin and hair and the transformation of body fluids into perspiration and urine are inseparable from the expanding, dispersing, cleaning-up, and pushing-downward functions of the lungs, which is why the lungs are considered the upper source of water.

Among the internal organs, the kidneys play a very important role in the production and metabolism of body fluids. This is because all the organs involved in body fluids depend on the warming and pushing power of the kidneys, including the stomach (which receives water), the spleen (which transports and transforms water), and the lungs (which spread and clean up water); in addition, the production and excretion of urine and the metabolism of water throughout the whole body are inseparable from the transforming function of the kidneys. This is why it is said that the kidneys are water organs and they take charge of the water throughout the entire body.

Insufficient body fluids and failure of water to transform into body fluids with water retention are the two basic pathological changes in metabolism of body fluids. Insufficient sources and excessive loss and consumption are the two basic causes of insufficient body fluids. The first cause may be due to insufficient intake of water and failure of water to transform into body fluids; the second may be due to the attack of a "hot" pathogen, excessive perspiration, vomiting, and diarrhea.

CAUSES OF DISEASES

The Six External Pathogens

The six external energies are wind, cold, summer heat, dampness, dryness, and fire, which stand for changes in climate during the four seasons. When these six external energies attack the human body through the mouth, nose, or skin to cause superficial disease, they are called the six external pathogenic energies, or the six external pathogens.

Wind   As one of the six external pathogens, wind can cause disease along with another external pathogen; so, a given disease may be caused by a combination of two pathogenic energies, such as wind-cold, wind-heat, wind-dampness, or wind-dryness. Wind is a yang pathogenic energy, and, when it causes disease, it will give rise to wandering symptoms and symptoms that change a great deal.

Wind can refer to external wind and internal wind. As one of the six external pathogenic energies, external wind attacks the human body from the outside. Internal wind, on the other hand, causes disease from within. When heat and fire reach their peaks, they may be transformed into internal wind; blood deficiency with yin exhaustion and energy and blood disturbances may also generate internal wind. The symptoms caused by internal wind include vertigo, fainting, twitching, trembling, numbness, and wry mouth and eyes.

Injurious wind refers to the disease caused by wind, normally called the common cold. In clinical practice, there are two types: common cold due to wind and cold, and common cold due to wind and heat. The two types are treated differently.

Cold   Cold is one of the yin external pathogenic energies that can easily cause harm to yang energy. When a person's yang energy is in deficiency, defense energy will fail to guard the body against foreign invasion; so, cold energy will attack, giving rise to such symptoms as dislike of cold, fever, headache, pain in the body, pain in bones and joints, and abdominal pain with diarrhea.

Like wind, cold can be divided into external and internal types. External cold refers to the cold energy that attacks the body from the outside. External cold causes a blockage of yang energy, with such symptoms as dislike of cold, fever, absence of perspiration, headache, pain in the body, and superficial and tight pulse. External cold can also refer to a weakening of yang energy in the body, with such symptoms as fear of cold and being very susceptible to an attack of the common cold. Internal cold refers to a weakening of yang energy, with a decline in organ functions that may give rise to disturbances of water transformation, retention of urine, and the like.

There can also be a direct attack of cold. Referred to as cold stroke, this is when the cold pathogenic energy attacks while the person is suffering from yang deficiency. The symptoms may include cold limbs and deep and fine or slow and tight pulse.

Summer Heat Summer heat is one of the yang external pathogenic energies. When summer heat attacks the body, it will give rise to such symptoms as headache, fever, thirst, mental depression, excessive perspiration, and forceful and rapid pulse. Summer heat can also cause great harm to body fluids, which in turn leads to such symptoms as fatigue, weak limbs, and dry mouth. In certain regions, when a great deal of dampness or humidity accompanies a prolonged summer, summer heat can attack the body along with dampness to cause such symptoms as congested chest, nausea, vomiting, and diarrhea.

Dampness Dampness is one of the yin external pathogenic energies. It has a turbid, heavy, and sticky nature, and it can obstruct the activities of energy transformation performed by the spleen.

There are internal dampness and external dampness, and they cause different symptoms. External dampness refers to the dampness outside the human body, such as on the ground, in the air, or of rain and dew. It may give rise to such symptoms as heavy sensations in the head as if being wrapped up by a wet towel, soreness in the back of the neck, congested chest, sore loins, tired limbs, and sore joints. Internal dampness refers to a stoppage of dampness within the body normally due to an inability of the spleen to transform dampness because of spleen yang in deficiency. When this occurs, the patient will display such symptoms as poor appetite, diarrhea, abdominal swelling, scant urine, yellowish complexion, edema in the lower limbs, light color of the tongue with a moist appearance, and soft and relaxed pulse.

Dryness Dryness can be divided into internal dryness and external dryness. Both internal dryness and external dryness (one of the six external pathogens) can cause exhaustion to yin fluids. Symptoms of external dryness include pink eyes, dry sensations in the mouth and nose, dry lips, pain in the ribs, dry cough, and constipation. With internal dryness, the exhaustion of internal yin fluids is mostly due to a later stage of hot diseases or the result of vomiting and diarrhea, excessive perspiration, excessive bleeding, or improper use of drugs. The symptoms of internal dryness consist of hot sensations as if heat were coming from the bones, mental depression, dry lips, dry tongue, dry skin, and dry and withered nails, which are symptoms of yin being harmed by heat.

Fire Fire, the sixth external pathogen, can cause the diseases called warm heat and summer heat. Fire is also one of the life forces transformed by yang energy into what is called physiological fire. There are different types of physiological fire, including monarch fire, minister fire, and lesser fire. Fire can also refer to a manifestation due to pathological change, which means that all kinds of external pathogenic energies, including the seven emotions (see below) and internal injuries, can transform into fire and turn into pathological fire.

In addition, fire can be differentiated into excess fire and deficiency fire. Excess fire is due to an excess of external pathogenic energies, which are mostly seen in acute hot diseases, with such symptoms as high fever, excessive perspiration, thirst, insanity, pink eyes, red complexion, discharge of blood from the mouth, nosebleed, red tongue, yellowish and dry coating of the tongue, and rapid and forceful pulse. Deficiency fire is due to an exhaustion of yin fluids, which is mostly seen in chronic wasting diseases, with such symptoms as being hasty, insomnia, seminal emission with erotic dreams, night sweats, cough with sputum containing blood, red tongue with scant coating, and fine-rapid or deficiency-rapid pulse.

The Seven Emotions
The seven emotions are joy, anger, worry, contemplation, sorrow, fear, and shock. The seven emotions can cause disease, and, conversely, disorders of the internal organs can cause the seven emotions. *The Yellow Emperor's Classics of Internal Medicine* states: Anger will force energy to move upward; joy will cause energy to relax; grief will cause energy to disperse; fear will cause energy to move downward; cold will cause energy to constrict; heat will cause a reduction of energy; shock will cause a disorder of energy; labor will consume energy; contemplation will cause energy to coagulate; anger will cause upsurging energy, and in severe cases, the patient will display the symptoms of vomiting blood and diarrhea containing undigested foods. Thus, anger will cause energy to move upward. When one is joyful, the energy will remain in harmony and the will is fulfilled so that nutritive and defense energies will flow smoothly.

"Thus, joy will cause energy to relax. When one is in grief, the heart connectives will become cramped, the lungs will be expanded with lobes lifted up, the upper burning space will be blocked up, and the nutritive and defense energies will be unable to disperse; as the hot energy is in the internal region, it will extinguish energy. Fear will cause a decline of pure energy; when pure energy is in decline, it will cause a blockage of the upper burning space; when the upper burning space is blocked up, the energy will move downward; when the energy moves downward, the lower burning space will be distended; thus, the energy stream stops. In contemplation, the heart focuses on something, the spirits have a place to return to, and the righteous energy stays put; thus, the energy becomes coagulated."

Foods and Fatigue
When foods cause disease, it is called a food injury. Intoxication, overeating, and eating foods with cold or cool energies are common causes. In addition, a prolonged consumption of greasy foods will cause a disorder of the digestive functions and produce internal heat and skin eruptions.

Fatigue is one of the factors that cause deficiency disease. The fatigue may be of an internal organ or due to excessive sex. Also called a bedroom injury, excessive sexual intercourse can harm the kidneys and become a chronic disorder.

THE INTERNAL ORGANS

The internal organs include the five viscera and the six bowels. The five viscera are the liver, heart, spleen, lungs, and kidneys. *The Yellow Emperor's Classics of Internal Medicine* states: "The heart is in tune with the blood vessels; its prosperity is manifest in the complexion; its master is the kidneys. The lungs are in tune with the skin; their prosperity is manifest in the hair; their master is the heart. The liver is in tune with the tendons; its prosperity is manifest in the nails; its master is in the lungs. The spleen is in tune with the muscles; its prosperity is manifest in the lips; its master is in the liver. The kidneys are in tune with the bones; their prosperity is manifest in the hair on the head; their master is the spleen." The word "master" refers to the controlling status in the five-elements theory, and the word "prosperity" means that when the internal organs are in good health, it will show on body surfaces, such as the hair or the ears or nose.

The six bowels refer to the gallbladder, small intestine, stomach, large intestine, bladder, and triple burning space. The following passage is from *The Yellow Emperor's Classics of Internal Medicine*. "The stomach, large intestine, small intestine, triple burning space, and bladder are the five organs generated by the energy of the Heaven, and their energies bear a resemblance to the energy of the Heaven. Thus, they drain off things without storing them up, they receive turbid energies from the five viscera, and they are called transmitting bowels. As they cannot store things up for long, they have to drain things off in due course. The door of physical strength (anus) also acts as the messenger for the five viscera and drains off water and grains without storing them up for long. The so-called five viscera are such that they store up pure energy without draining off, and, for that reason, they can be filled to capacity but cannot be oversupplied. The six bowels are such that they transmit things without storing them up, and, for that reason, they may be oversupplied but cannot be filled to capacity. The reason is that after foods enter through the mouth, the stomach will be full and the intestines will still be empty. Therefore, it is said that the bowels may be oversupplied but cannot be filled to capacity and that the viscera may be filled to capacity but cannot be oversupplied."

The Heart

The heart is the master of the human body and in control of human activities; it is in charge of various parts of the body and coordinates the functions of other internal organs, which is why the Chinese have a saying to the effect that "The heart is the master of the five viscera and the six bowels." The pericardium forms the external defense of the heart, and, for this reason, whenever a pathogenic energy tries to attack the heart, it must pass through the pericardium first. When the pericardium is under attack, it may give rise to such symptoms as high fever, coma, and delirium, which are considered the symptoms of a diseased pericardium.

The heart is the master of the spirits, which include mental conditions, consciousness, and thought. This accounts for the Chinese expression, "The heart is the grand master of the five viscera and the six bowels, and it is the residence of the spirits." When the heart is diseased, all related activities will be disordered, giving rise to such symptoms as insomnia, many dreams, forgetfulness, and even mental confusion, manifested in incoherent speech and thoughts.

The heart is the master of the blood vessels, and its glory is manifest in the face. The blood vessels are the channels through which the blood circulates. The reason that the blood can circulate through the blood vessels is due to the pushing power of the heart. Therefore, the Chinese believe that when energy circulates smoothly, blood will also circulate smoothly; on the other hand, when energy becomes sluggish, blood coagulations may result. The glory of the heart is expressed through a person's complexion, because when the heart is in good condition, the person's complexion will be shiny and reddish and manifest high spirits as well; conversely, when the heart is suffering from blood deficiency, the complexion will be pale and reveal low spirits.

The tongue is the outlet of the heart. The ancient Chinese believed that the heart extends its energy to the tongue; so, when the heart is in harmony, the tongue will be able to differentiate different flavors, which shows the close relationship between the heart and the tongue. The tongue is the external cavity of the heart, so a disease of the heart will be manifested in the tongue. For instance, when the heart is suffering from a deficiency of blood, the tongue will look pale; when the heart is suffering from blood coagulations, the tongue will be decomposed and have ulcers on it; and when the heart cavity is obstructed by sputum, stiffness of the tongue will occur. Therefore, two Chinese phrases are often mentioned in relation to the heart: "the heart with its cavity in the tongue" and "the tongue as the seedling of the heart."

The Small Intestine
The primary function of the small intestine is that of receiving water and grains from the stomach; it is in charge of transformation of foods and differentiating clear energy from turbid energy. When water and grains enter the small intestine from the stomach, they are further digested by the small intestine and the clear energy is absorbed; then they pass through the spleen to be transmitted to various parts of the body to become the material base of human activities. On the other hand, the turbid energy will be passed on to the large intestine and to the bladder for excretion.

The heart and the small intestine are connected to each other through meridians, and they form a yin-yang relationship with each other. The small intestine meridian is in the superficial region, whereas the heart meridian is in the deep region. When the heart meridian is suffering from excess fire, it will pass it on downward to the small intestine, causing such symptoms as short streams of reddish urine, burning sensations in the urethra, and pain or discharge of blood on urination, which should be treated by clearing the heart and promoting urination.

Two major syndromes of the heart are blood deficiency of the heart and yin deficiency of the heart. These two syndromes can be seen in general weakness, neurosis, and anemia, with the following symptoms: palpitations, depression, insomnia, many dreams, forgetfulness, and easily in shock. However, in cases of blood deficiency of the heart, the patient will more likely display pale complexion, pale tongue, and a deep and fine pulse, and, in cases of yin deficiency of the heart, low fever, night sweats, red zygoma, feeling depressed, hot and dry mouth, red tongue, and a fine and rapid pulse. Yin deficiency of the heart should be treated by toning up the yin of the heart, while blood deficiency of the heart should be treated by toning up the blood of the heart, and, for both, it is necessary to secure the spirits of the heart.

Energy deficiency of the heart and yang deficiency of the heart are also common syndromes of the heart. They can be seen in heart disease, heart failure, irregular heartbeats, neurosis, and shock. In cases of heart energy deficiency, there will be such symptoms as palpitations, shortness of breath, excessive perspiration becoming worse with labor or movements, fatigue, weakness, whitish complexion, congestion in the region before the heart, pale tongue with thin and white coating, and a fine and weak or clotting and slowing pulse. In cases of heart yang deficiency, there will be such additional symptoms as cold sensations and cold limbs; in cases of heart yang deficiency prolapse, there will be severe perspiration, coma, extremely cold limbs, and disappearing pulse about to exhaust. Heart energy deficiency should be treated by toning up heart energy, heart yang deficiency should be treated by warming up heart yang, and heart yang deficiency prolapse should be treated by restoring yang and fixing the prolapse.

The Liver
The liver is one of the most important internal organs in the human body, as it takes charge of storing and regulating the blood throughout the whole body and is also in control of flexing and extending joints and muscles. The liver loves to disperse and grow; it hates to be inhibited and oppressed. Therefore, when the liver is inhibited by the emotion of anger, it will be harmed as a result. For this reason, when the liver is diseased, the patient will display many emotional problems and disturbances. The liver has its outlets in the eyes and forms a yin-yang relationship with the gallbladder. The liver meridian travels around the yin organs (namely, the external genitals), passes through the lower abdomen, and spreads around the ribs, with the two branches meeting at the vertex. Thus, when disease occurs in the regions through which the liver meridian passes, the liver should be treated accordingly.

There is a well-known saying in Chinese medicine that goes like this: "The liver is in charge of storing the blood, and when a person lies down, the blood will return to the liver for storage. When the person becomes active again, the blood in the liver will flow to all parts of the body once again to meet the needs of various parts of the body."

The liver controls the activities of the tendons, ranging from extension and flexing of joints to nourishment of the tendons. When blood deficiency of the liver occurs, the tendons will suffer from malnutrition, which gives rise to difficulty in extension and flexing of joints, numbness, spasms, and the like. In addition, the nails will also change color and appear withered, because the nails are an extension of the tendons.

The eyes and the liver are very closely related to each other. When blood deficiency of the liver occurs, the eyes will suffer from malnutrition, giving rise to such symptoms as dry eyes, blurred vision, or night blindness. When liver-fire burning upward occurs, there will be the symptom of pink eyes. Many eye diseases are related to the liver and should be treated by reference to the liver.

The liver and the gallbladder form a yin-yang relationship with each other, as the liver is a viscus while the gallbladder is a bowel, and they are related to each other like brother and sister.

The Gallbladder

The gallbladder is attached to the liver and situated below the ribs. Although it is one of the six bowels, it differs from other bowels in that its bile is pure as opposed to other bowels that contain turbid substances. When the gallbladder is diseased, the following symptoms will occur: pain in the ribs, bitter taste in the mouth, vomiting of bitter water, and jaundice. As the gallbladder and the liver form a yin-yang relationship with each other, the diseases of the gallbladder are often treated by reference to the liver.

Liver and gallbladder dampness-heat is a well-established syndrome that can be seen in acute hepatitis with jaundice, acute cholecystitis, and gallstones, with the following symptoms: yellowish appearance of eyeball sclera, apparent pain in ribs, scant urine in reddish-yellow color, fever, thirst, nausea, vomiting, poor appetite, abdominal swelling, yellowish and greasy coating of tongue, and wiry and rapid pulse. To treat this syndrome, it is necessary to clear the heat, benefit the dampness, benefit the gallbladder, and reduce yellowish appearance.

The Spleen

The stomach receives foods and digests them, and then the spleen digests them for a second time, before sending them to the lungs to be transmitted to all parts of the body.

The most important energy of the human body is what is called "true energy," which is in close relationship with the spleen and the lungs. The spleen sends digested foods to the lungs to be mixed with the energy of the air inhaled by the lungs, and the two energies form the important ingredients of true energy. This is why the spleen is capable of producing energy. Therefore, when a person is suffering from energy deficiency accompanied by spleen deficiency, the function of the spleen in producing energy may have already been impaired and should be treated first.

The spleen governs the blood circulating throughout the entire body to prevent the blood from overflowing outside the blood vessels. Energy deficiency of the spleen may impair its function of governing the blood, resulting in various types of bleeding.

As spleen energy is capable of elevating, it can transport pure energy and pure substances of water and grains upward to the lungs and then to other internal organs to be transformed into energy and blood. If spleen energy fails to elevate and caves in instead, then symptoms such as shortness of breath, too tired to talk, chronic diarrhea, prolapse of the anus, prolapse of the uterus, and falling of other organs will occur, which are due to middle energy falling.

The spleen likes dryness and dislikes dampness. When the spleen fails to perform its functions of transformation and digestion due to its deficiency, it will generate dampness; conversely, excessive dampness will contribute to the difficulty of the spleen in performing its functions. When the spleen is being troubled by dampness, such symptoms as these will occur: heavy sensations of the head, feeling as if the whole body is sinking down, discharge of watery stools, and white and greasy coating of the tongue. For this condition, it is necessary to dry up the dampness and strengthen the spleen, and the herbs used should be relatively warm and dry.

The Stomach
The stomach performs the functions of receiving and digesting foods. It is also in charge of pushing down turbid substances. When stomach energy moves downward, water and grains will also move downward, which contributes to digestion, absorption, and excretion. If, instead of moving downward, stomach energy moves upward, then it will cause such symptoms as belching, hiccups, nausea, and vomiting.

The stomach likes dampness and dislikes dryness. It is very susceptible to the attack of heat, which is called the hot stomach syndrome. When heat attacks the stomach, it will cause harm to stomach fluids and cause such symptoms as dry tongue and mouth and thirst with craving for drink. To treat the hot stomach syndrome, it is necessary to nourish the yin of the stomach and produce fluids.

The spleen and the stomach form a yin-yang relationship, in that the spleen is a yin viscus while the stomach is a yang bowel. The spleen is in charge of elevation, whereas the stomach is in charge of downward movements; the spleen likes dryness, while the stomach likes dampness. They rely on each other in order to exercise control over each other in performing their respective functions of digestion and absorption.

Energy deficiency of both the spleen and the stomach is a distinct syndrome in Chinese medicine. This syndrome may be seen in ulcers, chronic gastritis, chronic enteritis, chronic dysentery, functional disorders of the stomach and intestine, tuberculosis of the intestine, chronic hepatitis, and cirrhosis of the liver, with such symptom as poor appetite, belching, swallowing of acid, nausea, vomiting, stomachache with desire for massage, pain getting better after a meal, fullness of stomach, abdominal swelling with discharge of watery stools, and edema. Should the disease become chronic, these symptoms will occur: withered and yellowish complexion, fatigue, weakness, loss of weight, light color of the tongue with white coating, fat and tender tongue with tooth marks appearing, and soft and weak pulse. To treat this syndrome, it is necessary to strengthen the spleen and harmonize the stomach.

Deficiency coldness of the spleen and the stomach is another common syndrome, called yang deficiency of both the spleen and stomach. It may be seen in ulcers, chronic gastritis, chronic enteritis, chronic dysentery, functional disorder of the stomach and intestine, edema, chronic hepatitis, and cirrhosis of the liver, with the following symptoms: abdominal pain, love of heat and warmth, full of clear saliva, hiccups, vomiting, poor appetite, abdominal swelling after meals, fatigue, weakness, cold limbs or scant urine, puffiness, whitish vaginal discharge, light color of the tongue with white-sliding or white-greasy coating, and a deep, fine, weak pulse. In treating this syndrome, it is necessary to warm and tone up both the spleen and the stomach.

Another common syndrome, called stomach-fire, may be seen in high-fever stages of various contagious diseases, diabetes, periodontitis, and mouth ulcers, with the following symptoms: thirst with craving for cold drink, periodic stomachache with burning sensations, red tongue, yellowish and thick coating of the tongue, dry tongue, and big and forceful pulse or sliding and rapid pulse. In order to treat this syndrome, it is necessary to clear and sedate stomach-fire.

Stomach yin deficiency also occurs and may be seen in chronic gastritis, gastric neurosis, indigestion, and diabetes, with the following symptoms: dry lips and mouth, lack of appetite, abdominal swelling after meals, discharge of dry stools, dry vomiting, hiccups, and dry tongue or burning pain in the stomach, red tongue with scant coating, and fine and rapid pulse. To treat this syndrome, it is necessary to nourish the yin of the stomach and clear the heat in the stomach.

The Lungs
The lungs are situated in the thoracic cavity and have the throat as their door and the nose as their outlet. They are a yin viscus, forming a yin-yang relationship with the large intestine, which is a yang bowel. The lungs are in charge of the respiratory energy, or the energy of air. When the lungs fail to control respiratory energy properly, they will give rise to cough, asthma, or difficult breathing.

After foods have passed through the stomach and spleen and been digested properly, they are mixed up with the clear energy of the lungs to become important ingredients of true energy for distribution throughout the entire body. When the lungs fail to distribute true energy properly, such symptoms as fatigue, weakness, shortness of breath, too tired to talk, and excessive perspiration will occur. These are all symptoms of the syndrome called energy deficiency of the lungs.

The lungs should be able to expand so that air can go through the nose and the mouth easily. When the lungs fail to expand, congested chest, cough, or asthma may occur. The lungs should also be able to push energy downward, and when they fail to do so, cough, asthma, scant urine, or edema may occur.

The lungs are in charge of opening and regulating waterways. Circulation of body fluids is a function of many organs working together as a team, including the lungs. Under normal circumstances, the lungs are capable of sending fluids downward to the kidneys, which pass the fluids to the bladder for excretion. When a pathogenic energy attacks the lungs to impair their normal functions, it will give rise to such symptoms as diminished urination and edema, which is why it is often said that "the lungs are the upper source of water."

The lungs are in charge of the voice, because the production of the voice and the functions of the lungs are closely related to each other. When the lungs are full of energy, the voice will be loud; when the lungs are suffering from energy deficiency, the voice will be feeble. Cold and wind may attack the lungs to cause energy congestion of the lungs, which will give rise to hoarseness or loss of voice.

The lungs use the nose as an outlet. The nose is the passage through which air comes and goes, so it is directly related to the lungs. When the lungs are functioning normally, air will go through the nose very smoothly and there will be a normal sense of smell. When the lungs are diseased, it will give rise to nasal congestion, nasal discharge, and an impaired sense of smell, and, in severe cases, there may be a flickering of the nostrils and difficult breathing.

The lungs are in charge of the skin and the hair. The skin and hair are the outermost regions of the human body, and the lungs can send defense energy and body fluids to them for nourishment. When the energy of the lungs is normal, the skin and hair will be moist and smooth and the pores will be well guarded. But as soon as the energy of the lungs becomes deficient, there will be a shortage of defense energy and the outermost regions will not be guarded properly, which will give rise to excessive perspiration and the common cold.

Both the lungs and the heart are situated above the diaphragm, with the lungs in charge of energy and the heart in charge of blood. When energy flows, the blood will circulate, and when energy congestion occurs, blood circulation will be impaired. Thus, the lungs and the heart can be seen to work together in control of energy flow and blood circulation.

The lungs are in charge of energy, and the spleen can produce energy. Thus, lungs diseases can, in many cases, be treated by toning up spleen energy. For example, a chronic cough with a great deal of white sputum can be treated this way.

The lungs and the large intestine form a yin-yang relationship with each other. Therefore, a cough and asthma due to excessive heat in the lungs can be treated by sedating the large intestine to clear up sputum heat, so the energy of the lungs will move downward, producing relief of the cough and asthma. And constipation, which is a symptom of the large intestine, may be due to energy deficiency of the lungs, in which case, the energy of the lungs should be strengthened to relieve the constipation.

The Large Intestine

The function of the large intestine is to excrete waste matter. When the large intestine is suffering from deficiency, it will cause constipation; when it is suffering from excess, it will cause diarrhea. Dampness-heat of the large intestine is a common syndrome often observed in acute bacillary dysentery, acute onset of chronic dysentery, and amoebic dysentery, with the following symptoms: abdominal pain, tenesmus, diarrhea with discharge of pus and blood, burning sensations in the anus, short streams of reddish urine, fever, yellowish and greasy coating of the tongue, and sliding and rapid pulse. In severe cases, there may be fainting and coma. In order to treat this syndrome, it is necessary to clear up heat and transform dampness in the large intestine.

The Kidneys

The kidneys are important organs in charge of growth, reproduction, and maintenance of the metabolic balance of water. Also, the kidneys are in charge of storing pure substances inherited from one's parents. Thus, the kidneys are innate roots of life. It is also believed that the formation of the fetus begins in the kidneys and that the two kidneys are formed prior to the body itself, so the kidneys can be seen as the roots of the viscera and the bowels as well as the 12 meridians. In clinical practice, some cases of slow growth of an innate nature are dealt with by treating the kidneys. Moreover, the kidneys are situated in the lumbar region, and, for this reason, it is said that the loins are the residence of the kidneys; so, when the kidneys are diseased, symptoms may occur across the loins. The kidneys include kidneys yin (true yin, or kidney water) and kidney yang (true yang, or life door–fire).

As already mentioned, the kidneys are in charge of storing pure substances, but "pure substances" refer to two different things. First of all, they refer to the pure substances of the five viscera and the six bowels derived from water and grains that have been digested and transformed by the spleen for distribution throughout the whole body, with extra-pure substances stored in the kidneys for future consumption. The pure substances also refer to those of the kidneys themselves, derived from the innate sources and mixed with the acquired energy of water and grains, which are closely related to the reproduction, growth, and aging of the human body. For this reason, when the pure substances of the kidneys are in short supply, a man may suffer from shortage of semen and infertility while a woman may suffer from suppression of menses and infertility, slow growth, and premature aging. All of these symptoms should be treated by toning up the kidneys.

The kidneys take charge of water. The regulation of body fluids is closely related to the following three organs: the lungs, spleen, and kidneys. This is called energy transformation of the triple burning space and was originally initiated by kidneys yang.

The kidneys are closely related to the growth and the softness or hardness of bones. For instance, in children, a fontanelle not closed after a long period of time can be dealt with by treating the kidneys; the same applies to soft bones in children and to the inability of an adult to stand up for very long due to weak legs. Teeth are extensions of bones, and loose teeth or teeth falling out are due to deficiency of kidney energy. The kidneys are in charge of storing pure substances, which generate marrow; marrow nourishes the bones and gathers in the brain. This is why it is said that the brain is the "sea of marrow." Kidneys energy deficiency, which is a common syndrome, may give rise to low intelligence, slow movements, and soft bones. In recent years, Chinese acupuncturists have applied the kidney point in auricular acupuncture to treat incomplete growth of the cerebrum in children and aftereffects of brain concussion, and the Chinese herbs that tone up the kidneys have been applied to treat aplastic anemia.

Under normal circumstances, the heart and the kidneys remain in balance, depending on each other as well as controlling each other, which is called mutual adjustment of yin and yang or communication between the upper organ and the lower organ. The heart yang is in the upper region, whereas the kidneys yin is in the lower region. The heart yang must rely on the kidneys yin for its supply of yin energy, while the kidneys yin must rely on the heart yang for its supply of yang energy. This interdependence is necessary in order to maintain normal functions of the human body and is called communication between the heart and the kidneys in Chinese medicine. When the heart or the kidneys are disordered, which disrupts the normal relationship between the two organs, insomnia, palpitations, forgetfulness, lumbago, and seminal emission can occur, which are the symptoms of the heart and the kidneys being incapable of communicating with each other.

The kidneys are also closely related to the liver. The liver is in charge of storing the blood, and the kidneys are in charge of storing pure substances. Pure substances and blood can generate and transform each other, which is why it is said that the liver and the kidneys originate from the same source. Under normal circumstances, kidneys yin will nourish and water liver yin. But when the kidneys are suffering from yin deficiency, the kidneys will be incapable of doing so, which will cause such syndromes as liver yin deficiency and liver yang upsurging. This is called water incapable of nourishing wood in the five-elements theory. On the other hand, yin deficiency of the liver will also cause yin deficiency of the kidneys. When both the liver and the kidneys are suffering from yin deficiency simultaneously, it is called yin deficiency of both the liver and the kidneys, which will cause such symptoms as lumbago, dizziness, and being hasty and jumpy.

The kidneys and the bladder are connected with each other through meridians. The condition of the energy of the kidneys has direct bearing on the capacity of the bladder in urination. This is why the kidneys and the bladder are said to form a yin-yang relationship with each other.

The Bladder
The bladder is in charge of storing urine and controlling urination. When the bladder is disordered, it will cause urination disorders and difficult urination. The reason that the bladder is capable of urinating is due to the energy transformation of the kidneys. When the energy transformation of the kidneys breaks down, difficult urination and retention of urine occur. And when the kidneys are suffering from deficiency, dribbling of urine and incontinence take place.

Bladder dampness-heat is a common syndrome observed in urinary infections, urinary calculus, and prostatitis, with the following symptoms: frequent urination, pain on urination or difficulty in urination, sudden interruption during urination, reddish-yellow and greasy coating on the tongue, and sliding and rapid pulse. To treat this syndrome, it is necessary to clear up heat and remove dampness.

The Pericardium
The pericardium is the protector of the heart; it is also its messenger. The pericardium is partially responsible for the symptoms of the heart, such as dizziness and delirium, which are normally considered symptoms of the pericardium as well. The heart is in control of the spirits, and it is the great master of the five viscera and the six bowels. When the heart is under attack, the patient will die due to its impact on the spirits; but, according to Chinese medicine, this doesn't happen very often, simply because before the pathogenic energy gets a chance to attack the heart itself, it must attack the pericardium.

The Triple Burning Space

The triple burning space refers to the three cavities in the human body, namely, the thoracic cavity (the upper burning space), the abdominal cavity (the middle burning space), and the pelvic cavity (the lower burning space). Why is it called the triple burning space? The reason is that this organ contains three parts, heats up the body, and is not really an organ but rather a cavity-like space.

According to *The Yellow Emperor's Classics of Internal Medicine,* "The triple burning space is the irrigation official who builds waterways." However, in performing this duty as the irrigation official, the triple burning space must cooperate with other internal organs, notably, the kidneys, bladder, and lungs. The kidneys and the bladder form a yin-yang relationship with each other, and the kidneys are connected with the lungs in the upper region. Thus, the triple burning space performs the irrigation duty in cooperation with the kidneys, lungs, and bladder, and particularly the lower burning space that excretes water into the bladder.

Disorders in the triple burning space may give rise to many urinary symptoms, including suppression of urination, dripping of urine, and edema. *The Yellow Emperor's Classics* states, "When the triple burning space suffers from an excess disease, it will cause anuria; when it suffers from a deficiency disease, it will give rise to enuresis." The same classic says, "The symptoms of the diseases of the triple burning space are as follows: congested abdomen, especially hardness in the lower abdomen; anuria that creates a desperate desire to discharge urine; and retention of urine that leads to an accumulation of water in the body and causes swelling."

According to another Chinese medical classic, when heat is present in the upper burning space, it will give rise to cough and pulmonary tuberculosis. According to still another classic, excessive heat in the upper burning space will cause perspiration on the forehead, abdominal swelling, pain in the rib region, dry tongue, scorching mouth, and blocked throat; coldness in the upper burning space will cause inability to eat, vomiting of acid, pain in the chest and back, affecting each other, and dry and sore throat.

When heat is present in the middle burning space, it will give rise to various types of dry and hard symptoms, such as constipation, abdominal swelling, and cough. When the middle burning space suffers from deficiency and cold, it will give rise to incessant diarrhea, indigestion, fullness in the middle, and intestinal swelling and rumbling.

When the lower burning space is deficient and cold, it will give rise to enuresis, incontinence of urination, and diarrhea. When the lower burning space suffers from excessive heat, it will give rise to discharge of urine containing blood, urination difficulty, suppression of urination, and difficult bowel movements.

The Brain, Marrow, and Womb

In addition to the viscera and the bowels, there are other organs, such as the brain, marrow, and womb, which are called the odd and constant organs, in distinction from the viscera and the bowels. Each type of organ performs a different function and, at the same time, is connected with the others and influences the others.

In addition to the brain, marrow, and womb, the odd and constant organs include bone, vessels, and the gallbladder. It seems that the gallbladder alone occupies a special status in the human body, as it is regarded both as a bowel (as mentioned earlier) and as an odd and constant organ.

The brain is the uppermost organ among the six odd and constant organs, and it is the material base of all mental activities. Therefore, the brain is also called "the organ of original spirit." The pathways in which the marrow travels upward and downward extend to the brain on the top and to the coccyx and sacrum at the bottom. This bears a resemblance to the conception of the central nervous system in modern Western medicine.

The brain and marrow are closely connected to the kidneys. The kidneys are in control of bones, bones generate marrow, and marrow travels through the brain, which is the "sea of marrow." Hence, when the pure energy of the kidneys is in abundance, the marrow in the brain will be in full supply and, consequently, one will be energetic and in high spirits. The womb in women is a synonym for the uterus, which exists for menstruation and nourishing the embryo and fetus. The function of the uterus is to some extent dependent upon the fullness of the pure energy of the kidneys.

DIAGNOSIS

The Four Methods of Diagnosis

The four methods of diagnosis refer to diagnosis by observations, questioning the patient, hearing and smell, and taking the pulse. In clinical practice, the four methods are used in combination.

Detecting internal conditions through external manifestations is the key to diagnosis in Chinese medicine. This is based upon the theory that any internal conditions will be manifest externally. Thus, a physician is able to know about the internal conditions of a patient through such external manifestations as complexion, skin conditions, and the spirits.

Diagnosis by Observations   In making a diagnosis through observations, the physician uses the power of his or her eyes to evaluate the patient's spirits, general physical condition (as manifest in muscles, bones, and skin), eyes, "outlets," complexion, and tongue. In the case of very young patients, fingerprint observation is also included.

Observations of the spirits are intended to determine whether the spirits are there, lost, or prolapsed. A person's spirits are present, or a person is in good spirits, when his or her eyes are active, speech is clear, complexion is moist and shiny, and breath is in balance. When a person is in good spirits, a disease can be more easily treated with better results. A person's spirits are lost when his or her eyes are passive, speech is incoherent, complexion is dull and dry, and breath is in imbalance. When a person is lacking spirits, a disease may prove more difficult to treat. Prolapse of the spirits refers to a deterioration of the loss of the spirits, which indicates a critical stage of a disease that should be treated as an emergency.

By observing physical conditions, such as of muscles, bones, and skin, a physician is able to know about the conditions of a patient's energy and blood. Observations of the spirits as expressed through the eyes can prove useful in understanding the conditions of energy and blood in the internal regions.

Observation of "outlets" is also important. "Outlets" refer to the outlets of the five viscera, namely, the tongue as the outlet of the heart, the nose as the outlet of the lungs, the eyes as the outlets of the liver, the lips as the outlets of the spleen, and the ears as the outlets of the kidneys. Observations of these outlets will enable a physician to understand the conditions of the corresponding viscus. For instance, a crimson tongue will indicate burning of heart-fire, blisters on the tongue will indicate dampness-heat in the spleen, and ringing in the ears will indicate an exhaustion of the kidneys. However, in making diagnosis, the whole body should be taken into consideration, and, for this reason, other aspects of diagnosis should also be taken into account.

Observing a patient's complexion includes evaluating whether the color is deep or superficial and dispersing or gathering, and whether the skin is moist or dry. Brightness is seen as a superficial color that indicates a superficial disease; darkness is viewed as a deep color that indicates a deep disease. A light and falling color is one that is dispersing, which generally indicates a new disorder involving the superficial region; a deep and accumulating color is one that is gathering, which usually indicates a chronic and severe disease. A moist appearance of the skin indicates the presence of stomach energy; a withered appearance indicates the decline of stomach energy.

The complexion of a normal person should be shiny and moist, with a mixture of yellow and red. The color of a normal complexion can also be seen in terms of host color and guest color. Host color refers to the base color that varies with individuals, while guest color refers to the color of the face that varies with the climate and other environmental or physical conditions. A normal complexion indicates normal conditions of the five viscera. Likewise, when a person has a very good complexion, it means that the energy conditions of the five viscera are excellent.

The complexion of a person can also be evaluated in terms of "good outlook" or "bad outlook." A moist and bright complexion indicates a good outlook, whereas a withering and dry complexion indicates a bad outlook.

As fingerprints are more visible in children than adults, a diagnosis by fingerprint can be used with children under three years old. Diagnosis by fingerprint focuses on the color and density of the print.

In making a diagnosis, a physician should use the thumb and forefinger of his or her left hand to hold the tip of the patient's forefinger, while using the thumb of his or her right hand to lightly push the patient's forefinger from the tip towards the base. This way, the print will become more visible.

The physician should observe the print very carefully. A normal fingerprint will appear reddish yellow with a degree of brightness. When the print appears to be floating, it normally points to a superficial disease; when it appears deep, it normally points to a deep disease. A light color of a fingerprint generally points to a deficiency or cold disease; a purple-red color to a hot disease; a blue-purple color to convulsions, wind-cold, pain, indigestion, and wind-sputum; and a black color to blood coagulations.

Observation of the tongue, commonly called tongue diagnosis, is an important aspect of diagnosis by observations. It primarily focuses on the coating of the tongue and the quality of the tongue with reference to shape, colors, movement, and degree of moisture. There is a Chinese saying that goes like this: "Differentiation of the quality of the tongue enables us to differentiate the five viscera regarding excess and deficiency; observations of the tongue coating enable us to determine how deep the six external pathogenic energies have penetrated into the human body."

The quality of the tongue is also called the body of the tongue. In evaluating the tongue, it is generally believed that the tip of the tongue is symptomatic of the heart and lungs, the sides of the tongue are symptomatic of the liver and gallbladder, and the root of the tongue is symptomatic of the kidneys. But these are only broad associations that should be applied with flexibility.

A moist tongue often indicates the presence of sufficient body fluids; a withered tongue often indicates an exhaustion of body fluids. An "old" tongue often indicates an excess disease; a tender tongue often indicates a deficiency disease. When the body of the tongue appears light red, fat, and tender, it may point to a yang deficiency; when the body of the tongue appears thin and bright red, it often indicates a yin deficiency. When the tongue is as shiny as a mirror with a coating, it points to yin deficiency of the liver and kidneys. When the tongue is swollen and painful, it points to excessive fire in the liver.

In terms of the tongue coating, a normal coating is white, but the tongue will have only a thin layer of white and clear coating, which is produced by stomach energy. A pathological white coating of the tongue is primarily due to wind, cold, and dampness, and it indicates a superficial disease. If the coating appears thin and glossy, it is mostly due to internal cold and dampness or external wind and cold. If the white layer of coating appears dry, it is due to a shortage of fluids. If the white coating occurs in a disease due to an attack of external pathogenic energies, then it generally indicates that these energies are beginning to transform into heat that may cause harm to fluids. A thick layer of white and glossy coating generally points to an excess of internal dampness; if the patient is also suffering from a superficial disease at the same time, it is due to external cold producing internal dampness. A thick layer of white and dry coating is due to heat-harming fluids with an inability of dampness to undergo transformation. A tongue with a white, glossy, sticky, greasy coating is mostly the result of internal sputum and dampness.

A yellow coating of the tongue indicates a hot disease, namely, the presence of the hot pathogenic energy in the internal region. A thin layer of yellow and glossy coating points to a dampness-heat disease, and, in a disease of external pathogenic energy, this coating points to the external pathogen transforming into heat in the internal region with fluids remaining unharmed. A thin layer of yellow and dry coating points to the hot pathogen harming yin fluids. A thick layer of yellow and glossy coating points to dampness-heat in the stomach and intestine. A thick layer of yellow and dry coating points to an accumulation of heat-harming fluids. And a yellow and greasy coating of the tongue indicates dampness-heat in the spleen and stomach, dampness-sputum, or indigestion.

Diagnosis by Questioning the Patient   This consists of questioning the patient regarding pain, time of onset, history, habits, and so on. Chinese physicians from the past developed 10 essential questions for this purpose, concerning (1) cold and hot sensations, (2) perspiration, (3) head and body, (4) urination and bowel movements, (5) eating, (6) chest, (7) hearing, (8) thirst, (9) pulse and color, and (10) the spirits. Subsequently, the ninth and tenth questions have been changed. The ninth question now concerns old diseases, and the tenth question the causes of diseases.

Diagnosis by Hearing and Smell   This includes hearing the patient's voice and the sounds of coughing, respiration, and so on, and smelling the patient's mouth and body. Some diseases may give rise to offensive smells, such as ulcers, tumors, or carbuncles. In some acute contagious diseases or in failure of the liver and kidney functions, there may be special smells to be detected. In addition, when a patient is suffering from heat in the lungs and stomach, he or she may have bad breath; this may also be the case when a patient is suffering from indigestion.

Pulse Diagnosis   Pulse diagnosis involves the use of three fingers to press the radial artery of the wrist, with the throbbing segment of the radial artery divided into three sections, namely, the distal section, middle section, and proximal section. To take the pulse is to determine the pulse rate, force, wave, and so on. Numerous pulses were discovered in ancient China, and about 28 pulses are in frequent use in clinical practice today.

The pulse can tell us about the nature of diseases. For instance, a superficial pulse is symptomatic of a superficial disease, a rapid pulse is symptomatic of a hot disease, and a slippery or sliding pulse is symptomatic of a sputum disease, indigestion, excess-heat disease, or pregnancy.

A normal pulse is also called a constant pulse, which is indicative of stomach energy, and it appears harmonious, slow, but forceful, neither too fast nor too slow, and at about four beats per act of respiration or 70 to 75 beats per minute. Children may display a faster pulse. Pulse rate may also be influenced by physical activities, climate, and other environmental conditions.

Abnormal pulse refers to any pulse other than a normal one. For example, a big pulse is an abnormal pulse, unless it is taken when a person is engaged in energetic activities.

The 28 pulses most frequently used in diagnosis include the following: depth-related pulses (1. superficial pulse and 2. deep pulse), frequency-related pulses (3. slow pulse and 4. rapid pulse) strength-related pulses (5. deficiency pulse, 6. excess pulse, 7. big pulse, and 8. small pulse), length-related pulses (9. long pulse and 10. short pulse), movement-related pulses (11. slippery pulse, 12. retarded pulse, and 13. wiry pulse), change-related pulses (14. abrupt pulse, 15. clotting pulse, and 16. intermittent pulse), and combination pulses (17. relaxed pulse, 18. full pulse, 19. disappearing pulse, 20. tight pulse, 21. soft pulse, 22. weak pulse, 23. drumming pulse, 24. persisting pulse, 25. shaking pulse, 26. hidden pulse, 27. dispersing pulse, and 28. empty pulse).

The Eight Syndrome Classifications

The eight syndrome classifications are yang syndrome, yin syndrome, superficial syndrome, deep syndrome, cold syndrome, hot syndrome, deficiency syndrome, and excess syndrome. Yin and yang are opposed to each other and indicate the different types of disease; superficial and deep are opposed to each other and indicate the regions of a disease; cold and hot are opposed to each other and indicate the nature of a disease; and deficiency and excess are opposed to each other and indicate the conditions of a disease. The superficial, hot, and excess syndromes are all yang syndromes; the deep, cold, and deficiency syndromes are all yin syndromes.

Yang syndrome   A disease that is acute, active, forceful, and progressive belongs to the yang syndrome, with such symptoms as red complexion, fever, love of cold, nervousness, dry and cracked lips, love of drinking, loud voice, love of talking, rough breath, and constipation. When a symptom belongs to the yang syndrome, the pulse is normally superficial, big, rapid, slippery, excessive, and forceful and the tongue is normally red in color with a yellowish and dry coating or even prickles.

Yin syndrome   A disease that is chronic, weak, quiet, and inhibitive belongs to the yin syndrome, with such symptoms as pale complexion, fatigue, heavy sensations in the body, cold limbs, low voice, quiet with dislike of talking, feeble breath, shortness of breath, decreased appetite, love of heat, long and clear streams of urine, and abdominal pain with desire for massage. In the yin syndrome, the pulse is normally deep, fine, slow, and weak and the tongue is normally light in color and fat and tender, with a moist and sliding coating.

Superficial syndrome   A disease that occurs in the skin and hair or in the external regions of the meridians belongs to the superficial syndrome.

Deep syndrome   A disease that occurs in the internal organs belongs to the deep syndrome. For instance, a warm or hot disease due to external causes with the pathogenic energy residing at the superficial region of the body belongs to the superficial syndrome; but when the pathogenic energy enters into the deep region to affect the energy and blood or the internal organs, it belongs to the deep syndrome.

Cold syndrome   This syndrome includes all diseases caused by cold pathogenic energy or by a decline in yang energy with yin excess. The symptoms may include low body temperature, pale complexion, withered spirits, fatigue, sleeping with legs curled up, love of warmth, fear of cold, cold abdominal pain that lessens with warmth, absence of thirst or thirst with a craving for hot drink, discharge of watery stools, clear and long streams of urine, pale tongue with a white and sliding coating, and deep and slow pulse, which are mostly seen in chronic and weak diseases.

Hot syndrome   This syndrome includes all diseases caused by hot pathogenic energy or an excess of yang energy. The symptoms may include fever, depressed feeling, red complexion, dislike of heat, dry lips and mouth, love of cold drink, red and dry lips, constipation, short streams of reddish urine, red tongue with a yellowish and dry or black and dry coating, and rapid pulse, which are usually seen in contagious and excess diseases.

32

Deficiency syndrome This syndrome encompasses all diseases caused by a decline in body energy. The symptoms of this syndrome include pale complexion, low spirits, fatigue, weakness, palpitations, shortness of breath, excessive perspiration, night sweats, tender tongue with no coating, and deficient and weak pulse.

Excess syndrome This syndrome encompasses all diseases caused by an excess of pathogenic energy engaged in a violent struggle with body energy or an occurrence of energy congestion and blood coagulations due to an internal functional breakdown that may also lead to sputum and indigestion. The symptoms of the excess syndrome may include high fever, thirst, mental depression, delirium, abdominal fullness and pain that worsen with massage, constipation, short streams of reddish urine, "old" tongue with a yellowish, dry, and rough coating, and excess and forceful pulse, which are mostly seen in acute diseases.

THE EIGHT GRAND METHODS OF TREATMENT

There are eight grand methods of treatment in Chinese medicine that have been established as the guiding principles in clinical practice. They are the methods of inducing perspiration, clearing heat, inducing bowel movements, striking a balance (or the harmonizing method), warming up coldness, tonification, eliminating, and inducing vomiting.

The Method of Inducing Perspiration

Inducing perspiration is also called initiating the superficial region in Chinese medicine. The objective of inducing perspiration is to induce the external pathogenic energies that have penetrated the human body to move outward by means of perspiration. In Chinese medicine, it is maintained that a pathogen will attack the human body from the outside and then it will penetrate into the body, step by step. For this reason, when the pathogen is still residing in the superficial region (namely, the regions of the skin, hair, and muscles), it is necessary to induce perspiration. This way, the pathogen will have a chance to get out of the body before it penetrates further into the body to cause a deep syndrome. The superficial syndrome, including such symptoms as dislike of cold, fever, headache, pain in the body, and superficial pulse, should be treated by inducing perspiration. As each patient is different in terms of physical conditions and as each disease is also different, the superficial syndrome is further divided into the superficial cold syndrome and the superficial hot syndrome. However, the two syndromes are, in most cases, closely related to each other, and, in clinical practice, they are usually treated together. Perspiration can be induced with pungent and *warm* herbs or with pungent and *cold* herbs.

In Chinese herbal therapy, herbs or foods with a pungent flavor and warm energy are used to treat a superficial cold syndrome, which displays the following symptoms: dislike of cold, fever, no perspiration, headache, nasal congestion, pain in the four limbs, thin and white coating of the tongue, and superficial and tight pulse or superficial and relaxed pulse.

In Chinese herbal therapy, herbs or foods with a pungent flavor and cold energy are used to treat the superficial hot syndrome, which displays these symptoms: fever, headache, slight dislike of cold and wind, presence of perspiration, thirst, sore throat, red tongue with a thin, yellow, and dry coating, and superficial and rapid pulse.

The Method of Clearing Heat

To clear heat means to clear and sedate the pathogenic heat for various kinds of deep and hot symptoms; clearing heat can also be used to treat deficiency heat or superficial heat. However, in clinical practice, a distinction must be made among the different types of heat, including energy heat, blood heat, yin heat, toxic heat, dampness-heat, heat in the internal organs, excess heat, and deficiency heat. For instance, energy heat and excess heat should be treated by clearing heat and sedating fire at the same time, blood heat should be treated by clearing heat and cooling the blood at the same time, yin heat should be treated by clearing the heat and nourishing the yin at the same time, toxic heat in excess should be treated by clearing heat and counteracting toxic effects at the same time, and heat in the internal organs should be treated by treating the organs involved.

To clear heat and sedate fire   Basically, this means treating energy heat, which normally displays the following symptoms: high fever, thirst, dry tongue, yellowish and dry coating of the tongue, and forceful and rapid pulse.

To clear heat and cool blood   This involves treating blood heat, which normally displays the following symptoms: high fever, mental confusion, delirium, deep-red tongue, and bleeding.

To clear heat and counteract toxic effects   This involves treating various types of toxic heat, which usually displays the following symptoms: red swelling, fever, pain, pustulation, and decomposition. Toxic heat includes the diseases caused by an attack of external energies, with such symptoms as sore throat, ulcers, vomiting of blood, nosebleed, and delirium, all of which belong to the hot syndrome.

To clear heat in the internal organs   This involves treating heat in the internal organs that display various symptoms. For instance, excess heat in the heart meridian will give rise to feeling depressed, thirst, ulcers in the mouth and on the tongue, short streams of reddish urine, difficulty in urination, and pain on urination; excess fire in the liver meridian will give rise to pain in the upper abdomen, bitter taste in the mouth, pink eyes and pain in the eyes, wax in the ears, urinary straining, ulcers in the genitals, and red swelling of the scrotum; heat in the lungs will give rise to cough and asthma; hot stomach or heat in the stomach will cause bad breath and swelling and bleeding of the gums, all of which may be treated by this method.

To clear heat and transform dampness   This involves treating dampness-heat, which generally displays the following symptoms: intermittent or prolonged fever, congested chest, abdominal swelling, sticky sensations in the mouth, nausea, poor appetite, reddish urine, watery stools, and yellowish and greasy coating of the tongue. The same method can also be used to treat a syndrome called dampness-heat turning into fire, which generally gives rise to dysentery, jaundice, hot urinary straining, or discharge of yellowish fluids in skin diseases.

To clear heat and lubricate dryness   This involves treating three syndromes: (1) the lungs-dryness syndrome, in which dryness impairs the lungs and the

34

stomach, causing dry throat, thirst, and dry cough with scant sputum; (2) the hot syndrome, particularly at its later stage when both energy and yin are impaired, causing such symptoms as dry mouth, mental depression, hiccups, and poor appetite; and (3) the deficiency heat syndrome, which gives rise to such symptoms as hot sensations in the body as if they were coming from the bones, periodic fever, night sweats, or persistent low fever.

The Method of Inducing Bowel Movements
Inducing bowel movements relieves constipation, and, for this reason, it can be used to treat a variety of syndromes as long as they involve constipation.

To sedate excess heat This method involves treating the following three syndromes: (1) The stomach-heat syndrome, with such symptoms as periodic fever, delirium, abdominal fullness, abdominal pain worsening with massage, constipation, scorching and yellowish coating of the tongue with prickles or scorching, black, dry coating on a cleft tongue, and slow and sliding pulse; (2) the toxic heat syndrome, with such symptoms as high fever, feeling depressed and hurried, mental confusion, twitching, dry mouth and throat, constipation, bleeding, and skin eruptions; and (3) heat in the internal organs, which gives rise to sore and swollen throat, ulcers in the mouth and on the tongue, swollen gums, nosebleed, bad breath, constipation, hot sensations in the chest and diaphragm regions, headache, pink eyes, ringing in the ears, feeling hurried and jumpy, and yellowish coating of the tongue.

To attack cold accumulations This method is used in treating the internal coldness syndrome. When a person consumes too much cold food with cold energy accumulating in the stomach and intestine, acute pain in the stomach and abdomen may occur that gets worse with massage. Or, when a person suffers from deficiency cold of the spleen and stomach, normal transformations and digestion are impaired, with the result that cold energy gets accumulated in the stomach and intestine, which may give rise to the following symptoms: abdominal pain that lessens with warmth, hardness felt with massage, thirst with craving for hot drink, constipation or difficult bowel movements, fear of the cold, cold limbs, and white and sliding coating of the tongue.

To lubricate the intestine to induce bowel movements This is used in treating the intestine-dryness syndrome for relief of constipation in older or weak patients or in pregnant women due to blood deficiency and shortage of fluids.

The Method of Striking a Balance, or Harmonizing
This method of treatment can also be called "negotiating a settlement," because it is aimed at regulating and adjusting the relationships among the internal organs, meridians, energy, and blood, for the purpose of removing external pathogenic energies to restore the normal functions of the body. This principle of treatment can be used in three different ways.

To harmonize the superficial and deep regions This involves treating the syndrome in between the superficial and deep, which normally displays the following symptoms: alternating cold and fever due to external causes, congested chest and discomfort in the upper-abdomen region, being quiet with no appetite, feeling depressed, nausea, bitter taste in the mouth, dry throat, dizziness, and wiry and rapid pulse.

To regulate and harmonize the stomach and the intestine This involves treating the cold and deficient large-intestine syndrome. When external pathogenic energies reside in the stomach and intestine, one may display such symptoms as combination of chills and fever, dull sensations at the pit of the stomach, nausea, abdominal pain, watery stools or diarrhea, and intestinal rumbling, which can be treated by this method.

To regulate and harmonize the liver and spleen or stomach This is used in treating two syndromes: the liver-spleen disharmony syndrome and the liver-stomach disharmony syndrome. The liver-spleen disharmony syndrome involves two distinct syndromes: the liver energy congestion syndrome and the spleen deficiency syndrome. The two syndromes are very similar and may include the following symptoms: feeling depressed, abdominal swelling and pain, discomfort in the chest, intestinal rumbling, and diarrhea or tension causing abdominal pain and diarrhea. The liver-stomach disharmony syndrome also involves two distinct syndromes: the liver energy congestion syndrome and the stomach energy upsurging syndrome. Likewise, both are very similar and may include such symptoms as congested chest, poor appetite, vomiting, belching, acid regurgitation, and pain at the pit of the stomach.

The Method of Warming Up Coldness

Warming up coldness is also called expelling coldness, and it is designed to tone up yang energy in order to expel the cold pathogen from the body. This method is used to treat the internal coldness syndrome, which is also called the deep coldness syndrome, as opposed to the superficial coldness syndrome. In Chinese herbal therapy, herbs to be used for warming up coldness are either warm or hot. The internal coldness syndrome is mostly due to a yang deficiency that has existed in one's physical conditions and generated coldness within the body or due to an attack of an external cold pathogen, resulting in a cold stroke, involving internal organs, that gives rise to a yang deficiency of the organs affected. Meridian coldness is mostly due to an accumulation of cold energy in the meridians causing a blockage of energy and blood within the meridians. There are a number of different methods of warming up coldness.

To warm the middle region and disperse coldness This involves treating the spleen-stomach yang deficiency syndrome, with such symptoms as cold pain at the pit of the stomach and in the intestine, vomiting, diarrhea, fat tongue with a white and sliding coating, and deep and slow pulse or deep and tight pulse; the spleen yang deficiency syndrome, with abdominal pain, love of warmth, abdominal swelling, watery stools, and cold limbs; and the cold stomach syndrome, with pain at the pit of the stomach that drags on and lessens with warmth or heat, vomiting of clear water, and more. In clinical practice, the spleen-stomach yang deficiency syndrome is encountered most frequently, as the spleen and the stomach form a yin-yang relationship with each other, so their symptoms will also affect each other.

To restore yang and rescue upsurging This is used to treat yang prolapse syndrome, with the following symptoms: dislike of cold, lying down with body curled up, extremely cold limbs, vomiting and diarrhea, body temperature decreasing, pale complexion, and fine and disappearing pulse or hollow and rapid pulse.

To warm up meridians and disperse coldness   This is designed to treat the meridian coldness syndrome, with the following symptoms: cold pain in the four limbs, poor blood circulation, blue tips of the four limbs, rheumatism with coldness, cold pain in the muscles, and difficulty in flexing and extending the joints.

The Method of Tonification
This treatment principle is an important one in Chinese medicine, as it can be applied to deal with inherent deficiency and acquired deficiency alike, so long as there are signs of yin or yang deficiency, energy deficiency, blood deficiency, shortage of semen, or shortage of fluids, and so on. There are four methods of tonification: to tone up energy deficiency, blood deficiency, yin deficiency, and yang deficiency.

To tone up energy deficiency   This involves treating the energy deficiency syndrome, the lungs energy deficiency syndrome, and the spleen energy deficiency syndrome. These syndromes may give rise to the following symptoms: fatigue, weakness, shortness of breath, too tired to talk, feeble and low voice, asthma triggered by labor or movements, whitish complexion, poor appetite, watery stools, excessive perspiration, edema, weak pulse, prolapse of the anus, and prolapse of the uterus.

To tone up blood deficiency   This is used to treat the blood deficiency syndrome, with the following symptoms: pale or withering and yellowish complexion, pale lips and nails, dizziness and spots in front of the eyes, palpitations, insomnia, irregular menstrual periods, scant menstrual flow in light color, numbness of hands and feet, pale tongue, and fine pulse.

To tone up yin deficiency   This is used to treat the yin deficiency syndrome, with the following symptoms: loss of weight, dry mouth and throat, dizziness, ringing in the ears, sore loins and weak legs, red tongue with scant coating, and fine pulse. The same treatment principle is also effective for the deficiency fire syndrome, with the following symptoms: red lips, reddish appearance in the zygoma, feeling depressed, insomnia, hot sensations in the middle of the palms and the soles of the feet, periodic fever, night sweats, seminal emission, and discharge of blood from the mouth.

To tone up yang deficiency   This is used to treat the yang deficiency syndrome, with the following symptoms: fear of cold, cold limbs, sore loins, weak legs, cold pain across the loins or in the legs, impotence, sliding ejaculation, a long stream of plentiful clear urine, pale tongue, and deep, fine, and weak pulse. All of these symptoms are mostly seen in the *kidneys* yang deficiency syndrome. The *heart* yang deficiency syndrome and the *spleen* yang deficiency syndrome should be treated by the principle of warming up.

The Method of Eliminating
This method of treatment is for such disorders as indigestion, swelling, accumulation, stones, ulcers, and parasites. It can be broadly divided into two categories: to eliminate hardness and to eliminate coagulations.

To eliminate indigestion This treatment principle is designed to cope with symptoms arising from indigestion as follows: fullness of stomach, abdominal swelling, acid swallowing and belching of bad breath, nausea, vomiting, poor appetite, abdominal pain, constipation, diarrhea, and thick and greasy coating of the tongue.

To eliminate swollen lumps and expel stones This principle can be applied in treating swollen lumps, such as of the liver and the spleen, and hard symptoms and tumors as well as liver stone, gallstone, urinary stone, and so on.

To eliminate carbuncles and drain off pus This principle is designed for such external infections as carbuncles, abscesses, boils, and furuncles. In clinical application, a further distinction between the yang syndrome and the yin syndrome is made. The yang syndrome includes the following symptoms: acute onset, redness, swelling, heat, pain, and sticky fluids in cases of ulcers. The yin syndrome includes slow onset, white and spreading swelling, hardness with aching pain, and clear and thin fluids in cases of ulcers.

To eliminate sputum and soften up hardness This principle can be applied to deal with hard sputum in the meridians, with the following manifestations: lipoma, fibroma, tuberculosis lymph node, goitre, nodular goitre, carcinoma of the thyroid, simple goitre, and so on.

The Method of Inducing Vomiting
Of the eight grand methods of treatment, inducing vomiting is the last. It is used to prevent poisoning and suffocation, consumption of toxic foods, presence of indigestible substances in the stomach, apoplexy, and epilepsy.

HERBOLOGY

In Chinese medicine, diseases are often treated with herbs. Applications of Chinese herbs in clinical practice are based upon the nature and capabilities of herbs, and they in turn are based upon the energies, flavors, movements, and meridian routes of herbs.

The Four Energies
The four energies of herbs are cold, hot, warm, and cool. These classifications are derived from the effects of herbs as originally observed from actual applications by the ancient Chinese. When an herb has proven effective in the treatment of a hot syndrome, that herb is considered to have a cold energy; when an herb has proven effective in the treatment of a cold syndrome, it is considered to have a hot energy. The four energies of herbs can be broadly divided into yin and yang, with cold and cool energies belonging to yin and hot and warm energies belonging to yang. Since the difference between cold and cool and between hot and warm is only a matter of degree, Chinese physicians are in the habit of using such expressions as "extremely warm" or "slightly warm" and "extremely cold" or "slightly cold."

The Five Flavors
The five flavors refer to pungent (or acrid), sweet, sour, bitter, and salty, which are distinguished from each other by the sense of taste. The ancient Chinese

distinguished various actions of herbs through a very long process of clinical experience, and they came to the conclusion that pungent herbs can disperse, sour herbs can constrict, sweet herbs can slow down, bitter herbs can harden, and salty herbs can soften up. This was clearly recorded in *The Yellow Emperor's Classics of Internal Medicine*. Subsequently, Chinese physicians have further discovered that pungent herbs can disperse and promote the flow of energy, sour herbs can constrict and obstruct, sweet herbs can tone up and harmonize, bitter herbs can dry up and cause diarrhea, and salty herbs can soften up and promote downward movements. In addition, there is another classification called tasteless flavor, which can help dampness seep and promote urination. But, as tasteless flavor is similar to sweet flavor, the two are generally classified under the same flavor, which is why a celebrated Chinese herbalist has said, "Tasteless flavor is associated with sweet flavor."

The Four Movements
The four movements of herbs are to push upward, to push downward, to float, and to sink. To push upward means that a given herb is capable of elevating falling symptoms, as with the prolapse of the anus and uterus or the internal organs. To push downward means the herb is capable of suppressing upsurging symptoms, as with hiccups and cough. To float means that the herb is capable of dispersing outward, as with inducing perspiration. And to sink means that the herb is capable of promoting diarrhea and directing energy downward. The herbs that can push upward and those that can float have the common functions of moving upward and outward, with such actions as inducing perspiration and vomiting as well as elevating yang energy. On the other hand, the herbs that can push downward and those that can sink have the common functions of moving downward and inward, with such actions as relieving vomiting, checking perspiration, and inducing diarrhea.

Meridian Routes
The meridian routes refer to the meridians a given herb is capable of entering and travelling through, which accounts for two herbs with identical energy and flavor still displaying two different actions. In clinical application, herbs are selected that travel through the meridians in the diseased regions. For instance, a hot herb is used to treat a cold disease and a cold herb is used to treat a hot disease, which are standard procedures in Chinese herbal therapy. But two hot herbs may have different actions, with one herb being good for the cold *lungs* syndrome while the other being good for the cold *liver* syndrome. By the same token, one cold herb may be good for the hot *spleen* syndrome whereas another cold herb may be good for the hot *lungs* syndrome.

Actions
All important Chinese herbs or herbal formulas have a number of common actions, which is why they are considered important. In Western medicine, an antihistamine is used to counteract the effect of histamine, which is the action of an antihistamine. Similarly, Chinese herbs or herbal formulas have various actions,

but they are expressed in different terminologies, such as to clear heat, sedate fire, or stop wind. The terminologies used for treatment principles and actions are identical. Thus, when a given formula can clear heat, its action is to clear heat, which may be used to treat the hot syndrome.

A formula may have, say, four common actions: to clear the lungs, transform sputum, cool the blood, and counteract toxic effects. A doctor of Chinese medicine knows how to use this formula simply by identifying its common actions. Since this formula can cool the blood, we can use it to arrest bleeding, as in the case of nosebleed; since it can clear the lungs, we can use it to suppress cough associated with the lungs; since it can transform sputum, we can use it to reduce mucous discharge in cough and asthma; and since it can counteract toxic effects, we can use it to heal swelling and boils in the skin.

Thus, the common actions of Chinese formulas are very important in clinical applications, but it takes quite a while for a person to fully understand the meaning of the common actions of formulas and learn how to apply them in the treatment of diseases. The basic reason is that in order to make use of common actions of formulas, one needs to know how to make diagnosis of a disease, which is not a very easy task. Even if we know, for example, that this particular formula can cool the blood, we still have a long way to go before we are able to apply it to arrest bleeding.

There are many possible syndromes that account for bleeding, including the wind-cold syndrome, the spleen unable to govern the blood syndrome, external injuries, the large-intestine excess syndrome, and the hot blood syndrome. If a formula can cool the blood, it can only be applied to treat nosebleed that falls within the scope of the hot blood syndrome in order to be effective. A doctor of Chinese medicine must make a diagnosis to determine if this particular case of nosebleed, for example, falls within the scope of the hot blood syndrome, before he or she can apply it to treat nosebleed. In addition, in order to determine the right syndrome of a nosebleed, the doctor needs to follow the standard procedures of Chinese diagnosis, which involve the theory of yin and yang as well as the Chinese organ theory.

Herbal Formulas

In most cases, a syndrome has more than one symptom that cannot be treated by one single herb. Thus, in Chinese herbal therapy, several herbs are used together in a formula in order to cope with the conditions of a disease. This is called compound therapy in Chinese medicine. Over the course of history, the Chinese have established more than 20,000 formulas, of which about 2,000 are currently in use. Although a physician of herbal therapy can use his or her own formulas to treat patients, established formulas have been proven effective in the past, and, for this reason, they should be used for clinical applications whenever possible.

A standard herbal formula consists of a king herb, subject herb, assistant herb, and servant herb. According to *The Yellow Emperor's Classics of Internal Medicine,* "The primary herb in a formula is called the king herb, the herb included in the formula to assist the king herb is called the subject herb in that formula, and the herb included in the formula to be responsible to the subject herb is called the servant herb."

Every formula must have at least a king herb, but not every formula needs a subject herb, an assistant herb, or a servant herb. Sometimes a formula may have a king herb that also plays the role of a subject herb, just like a prime minister may also act as the finance minister in a cabinet. As a general rule, the king herb in a formula has the largest dose, followed by the subject herb, the assistant herb, and the servant herb.

The king herb In a formula, the king herb is the herb that is primarily responsible for dealing with the syndrome under treatment. For instance, if the patient has been diagnosed as suffering from the cold syndrome, the king herb must be capable of warming up the body; if the patient has been diagnosed as suffering from the kidneys yang deficiency syndrome, the king herb must be capable of toning up the kidneys yang. Many formulas have more than one king herb, because a syndrome often contains two basic conditions that need to be treated simultaneously with two different herbs. Take the gallbladder dampness-heat syndrome for example. This syndrome contains two basic conditions, namely, gallbladder-dampness and gallbladder-heat, so the formula selected to treat this syndrome may contain one herb to remove gallbladder-dampness and a second herb to clear gallbladder-heat.

The subject herb An herb in this category assists the king herb in two different ways: it reinforces the action of the king herb from a different angle, and it treats the concurrent syndrome. For example, when the king herb in a formula is used to induce perspiration, a subject herb can be selected to produce body fluids to reinforce the function of the king herb in inducing perspiration. Sufficient body fluids will make perspiration easier, which means that the subject herb is helping the king herb achieve its objective indirectly. Another example is that when a person is suffering from two syndromes simultaneously, with one syndrome as the main one and the other syndrome as the concurrent one, the king herb will deal with the main syndrome while the subject herb will deal with the concurrent syndrome. As with king herbs, a formula can contain more than one subject herb.

The assistant herb In a formula, the assistant herb can play one of the following three roles: it can assist the king herb or the subject herb in dealing with a relatively minor symptom, it can control the undesirable drastic actions of the king herb and the subject herb or reduce their toxic effects, and it can play the role of an opposition to supplement the action of the king herb.

The servant herb In a formula, the servant herb plays two basic roles: it can direct the formula to the affected region, and it can harmonize the herbs in the formula.

How to Take Herbs
After herbs are put together in a formula, they must be prepared for consumption. There are three common ways of taking a formula: decoction, powder, and tablets.

Decoction As many Chinese formulas have been made into tablets and many are also available in powder form, it has become less important for people to know how to decoct formulas. Nevertheless, the vast majority of Chinese formulas are still not available in either tablets or powder, which means that they need to be decocted. Moreover, herbal formulas that have been decocted are readily absorbed and take effect more quickly, which is beneficial for acute disorders. In order to produce the best therapeutic effects, formulas should be decocted according to established methods.

The pot used for decoction should be made of something other than iron or bronze in order to prevent chemical changes; usually, an earthenware pot is used instead. Place the herbs in the pot, add cold water just enough to cover all the herbs, and then add one more cup, so that the water will be about half an inch higher than the herbs. Stir a little bit, and let the herbs soak in the water for about 20 minutes. Then bring the water to boil; as soon as the water begins to boil, reduce the heat to low, both to keep the water from overflowing and to prevent its premature exhaustion. During the course of decoction, the pot should be covered and not opened too frequently in order to retain the volatile constituents of some herbs. The quantity of the water used varies with the herbs and the heat, because some herbs absorb more water than others and thus need more water for decoction and high heat consumes more water than low heat.

Before decoction, herbs should be soaked in water for about 20 minutes to make them soft and moist. The same water should be used for decoction to prevent any loss of the herbs' potency. The total decoction time depends upon the herbs being decocted. For instance, herbs for inducing perspiration can be decocted over high heat for less than 10 minutes after the water starts boiling and herbs for strengthening the body, traditionally called tonics, can be decocted for as long as an hour over low heat. After decoction, the herbs are strained.

When a Chinese patient gets a prescription from a doctor, he or she usually brings it to an herb shop for filling. The clerk at the herb shop will wrap up the herbs in small paper bags and give instructions for each bag to be decocted two to three times for oral administration. Normally, each decoction is to be taken all at once as one dosage, usually in one or two cups, and two dosages are taken a day. The same bag of herbs can be decocted in the morning and then again in the late afternoon.

Sometimes it may be necessary to decoct the heavy or hard herbs, like wood or roots, over low heat for 10 to 20 minutes first, so that their constituents will become fully soluble in boiling water. Clinical experiences have shown that such heavy herbs can be decocted repeatedly to produce good results. After heavy and hard herbs have been boiled for 10 to 20 minutes, add the aromatic herbs and then the very light herbs, such as leaves and flowers, which should be decocted for only about five minutes or so in order to prevent evaporation of some constituents like essential oils.

Powder   When herbs in a formula are ground into powder, they are easy to carry, take, and preserve. Powder is also more economical than by decoction, because generally one bag of herbs supplying one day's consumption by decoction will supply four days of consumption in powder with the same effects. After the herbs have been ground into powder, filter the powder to make sure that it is fine enough for consumption. Here is how to take a formula in powder:

- The first thing you should do is mix up the powder thoroughly either in a jar or a bag to make sure that the powder is properly mixed, because herbal formulas contain different herbs which should be mixed up evenly.
- Put the powder in a cup, and pour boiling water into the cup; then stir and drink it warm. If any residue remains at the bottom, repeat the same process and drink it again, so that you don't waste any powder.
- The quantity of powder you should take depends on how much you weigh, because the heavier you are, the more you should take. Assuming that you weigh 140 pounds, you should be taking 6 grams of powder (roughly one-third of the formula weight) each time (increase or decrease 1 gram for each 15 pounds of body weight). Therefore, if you weigh 155 pounds you should take 7 grams each time; if you weigh only 110 pounds, you should take only 4 grams each time, twice daily.
- The process of drinking Chinese herbal powder is similar to drinking instant coffee, except the powder may not dissolve in boiling water as quickly and easily as instant coffee and the powder may not taste as good as coffee. If you don't like the taste of it, you can also put it in empty capsules, which are available in health food stores. Alternatively, you can place the powder on your tongue, hold your breath, and wash it down with a cup of warm water. Wash any residue down with another cup of water. This should be done twice daily.

Tablets Herbal powder can be made into tablets, which is normally done by manufacturers. Tablets have a number of advantages: they are easiest to take and carry; they are slow in absorption and therefore good for chronic and deficient diseases; and, since some formulas are very drastic in action, when they are taken as tablets, such drastic action can be slowed down. Follow the manufacturer's instructions on the quantity of tablets to take each time.

The Three Rules for Taking a Formula
There are three types of rule regarding taking an herbal formula, those specifying when the formula should be taken, whether it should be taken warm or cold, and that it should be taken without tea.

When to Take a Formula A formula can be taken before or after meals, depending on the formula and its effects. As a general rule, formulas that can disturb the digestive system and formulas for eye diseases should be taken after meals; formulas for malaria should be taken two hours prior to onset; formulas to induce sleep, as in insomnia, should be taken before bedtime; formulas for acute symptoms can be taken any time; formulas for chronic diseases should be taken according to a fixed schedule on a regular basis; and formulas taken as tonics to strengthen the body should be taken before meals. In addition, some formulas can be drunk like tea many times during the day without any fixed schedule.

The Chinese have this saying: "Withered plants will blossom and migratory birds return every year on schedule." When this principle is applied to taking formulas, it means that formulas should be taken regularly according to a fixed schedule or every day at the same time.

When formulas are used to treat disorders in the chest or above the chest, they should be taken after meals; when they are used to treat disorders below the heart, they should be taken before meals; when they are used to treat disorders of the four limbs and the blood vessels, they should be taken on an empty stomach; and when they are used to treat disorders of bones and marrow, they should be taken at night and after meals.

Whether the Formula Should Be Taken Warm or Cold   Some formulas should be taken very warm, but others taken cold, depending on the disorder under treatment. Formulas taken to induce perspiration, as for the common cold, should be taken very warm or relatively hot. The patient should keep warm right after taking the formulas in order to induce light perspiration, and, after taking such formulas, it is also wise to drink a little hot soup to reinforce the effects of the formulas.

When formulas are taken to treat a hot disease, they should be taken cold; when formulas are taken to treat a cold disease, they should be taken hot. However, certain formulas can cause vomiting when taken hot, in which case they should be taken cold.

Taking the Formula Without Tea   The third rule regarding taking formulas is to refrain from taking them with tea. Some people have a habit of taking formulas with tea for the sake of convenience, but this is definitely not advisable; warm water should be drunk instead. For one thing, tea is obstructive, and it can obstruct the movements of herbs, reducing their effects. In the second place, tea has a cold energy, which can interfere with the warm energy of certain herbs. And thirdly, tea contains caffeine and theophylline, which can excite the central nervous system; so, when formulas used to treat insomnia, for example, are taken with tea, their effects will be cancelled out.

ACUPUNCTURE

Although acupuncture and herbology are two different branches of Chinese medicine, with the former treating diseases by external methods and the latter by internal administration of herbs, they are frequently used simultaneously in clinical practice. Both are also based upon the theories of yin and yang, the five elements, the internal organs, and the meridians. In addition, both are guided by the four methods of diagnosis and the eight classifications of disease.

CLINICAL DIAGNOSIS

What follow are a few clinical cases presented for making a diagnosis to illustrate how you can use this book for self-healing purposes. In each case, key symptoms are in boldface to indicate that they should be checked against the symptoms listed under the headings of Headache (pages 48–51) or Hyperthyroidism (pages 119–121), depending on the chief complaint. All the syndromes under the headings are taken into account, and the ones with the highest score are used for diagnosis.

Clinical Case No. 1
Name of patient: Chen
Sex: male
Age: 29
Chief Complaint: headache
History and symptoms: The patient was **hit by a falling object** from the second floor while at work. He fainted on the spot and was sent to the hospital for treatment. On examination, he was found to have suffered skin injuries on the head and was experiencing sensations of aching pain. He was treated accordingly. Two weeks later, **prickling pain** occurred on the right side of the head that came in three or four attacks a day, worsening at night.

To make a diagnosis of headache as the chief complaint, a total of nine syndromes should be taken into account, as can be seen on pages 48–51.

The symptoms in boldface are to be checked against those listed under each of the nine syndromes. The symptoms in boldface are found under "9. Blood coagulations syndrome." So, the diagnosis can be presented as follows:

1. Wind-cold syndrome (0)
   None
2. Wind-heat syndrome (0)
   None
3. Wind-dampness syndrome (0)
   None
4. Liver yang upsurging syndrome (0)
   None
5. Dampness-sputum syndrome (0)
   None
6. Energy deficiency syndrome (0)
   None
7. Blood deficiency syndrome (0)
   None
8. Kidneys energy deficiency syndrome (0)
   None
9. Blood coagulations syndrome (5)
   Headache caused by external injuries (4)
   Prickling pain in the head (1)

Thus, the diagnosis is 9. blood coagulations syndrome, which has the highest score of 5.

Clinical Case No. 2
Name of patient: Zhou
Sex: female
Age: 36
Chief complaint: headache
History and symptoms: The patient has suffered **migraine headaches** since she was six years old and for more than 30 years. The **headache worsens with labor, fatigue, or use of the brain (thinking)**. The pain also gets worse each month during her menstrual period, which often occurs in a heavy flow, with **dizziness**, forcing her to lie down in bed for two or three days. Other symptoms include whirling sensations in the eyes, **palpitations**, poor memory, **withered complexion**, pale appearance of lips and nails, **fatigue,** and dislike of talking.

To make a diagnosis of headache as the chief complaint, a total of nine syndromes should be taken into account, as can be seen on pages 48–51.

The symptoms in boldface are to be checked against the symptoms listed under each of the nine syndromes.

1. Wind-cold syndrome (2)
   Dizziness (1)
   Headache with dizziness (1)
2. Wind-heat syndrome (2)
   Dizziness (1)
   Headache with dizziness (1)
3. Wind-dampness syndrome (0)
   None
4. Liver yang upsurging syndrome (8)
   Dizziness (1)
   Headache (1)
   Headache in women (1)
   Headache on the side of head (migraine headache) (5)
5. Dampness-sputum syndrome (5)
   Dizziness (1)
   Headache with dizziness (3)
   Prolonged dizziness (1)
6. Energy deficiency syndrome (6)
   Dizziness (1)
   Fatigued eyes and spirits (fatigue) (1)
   Headache that occurs on fatigue after labor (2)
   Prolonged headache (2)
7. Blood deficiency syndrome (5)
   Dizziness (1)
   Fatigue (1)
   Headache with dizziness (3)
8. Kidneys energy deficiency syndrome (3)
   Dizziness (1)
   Fatigue (1)
   Prolonged dizziness (1)
9. Blood coagulations syndrome (0)
   None

Thus, the diagnosis is 4. Liver yang upsurging syndrome, which has the highest score of 8.

Clinical Case No. 3
Name of patient: Jia
Sex: female
Age: 26
Chief complaint: hyperthyroidism
History and symptoms: The patient was diagnosed with hyperthyroidism at a hospital of Western medicine. She came to the clinic later with **palpitations, excessive perspiration, jumpiness, fear of heat, hot sensations in hands and feet, increased appetite, fatigue, low fever, dry mouth, poor sleep**, and **feeling as if some objects were in her throat.**

To make a diagnosis of hyperthyroidism as the chief complaint, a total of six syndromes should be taken into account, as can be seen on pages 119–121.

The symptoms in boldface are the symptoms to be checked against those listed under the six syndromes.

1. Hot stomach syndrome (2)
   Getting hungry easily (1)
   Thirst (1)
2. Liver energy congestion syndrome (5)
   Insomnia (1)
   Psychological tension (jumpiness) (2)
   Subjective sensations of objects in the throat (2)
3. Sputum-fire syndrome (14)
   Dislike of heat (3)
   Eat a lot (2)
   Emotionally disturbed easily (3)
   Excessive perspiration (2)
   Palpitations (3)
   Sleeplessness (1)
4. Liver-kidneys yin deficiency syndrome (5)
   Fatigue (3)
   Palms of hands and soles of

feet are both hot (1)
Sleeplessness with forgetfulness
(1)
5. Deficiency fire syndrome (9)
   Becoming angry easily (2)
   Excessive perspiration (2)
   Dry sensations in the mouth (1)
   Hot sensations in hands and
   feet (2)
   Low fever (1)
   Sleeplessness (1)
6. Simultaneous deficiency of yin
   and energy syndrome (8)
   Excessive perspiration (1)
   Fatigue (3)
   Hot sensations in hands and
   feet (1)
   Palpitations (2)
   "Tidal" fever in the after-
   noon (1)

Thus, the diagnosis is 3. Sputum-
fire syndrome, with the highest score
of 14.

Clinical Case No. 4
Name of patient: Li
Sex: female
Age: 38
Chief complaint: hyperthyroidism
History and symptoms: The patient
came to the clinic with
hyperthyroidism as diagnosed at a
hospital of Western medicine. She
displayed the following symptoms:
palpitations, excessive perspiration,

**misty vision, jumpiness, shaking of
hands, good appetite with frequent
hunger, weight loss, diarrhea, and
fatigue.**

To make a diagnosis of
hyperthyroidism as the chief
complaint, a total of six syndromes
should be taken into account, as can
be seen on pages 119–121.

The symptoms in boldface are the
symptoms to be checked against
those listed under the six syndromes.

1. Hot stomach syndrome (1)
   Getting hungry easily (1)
2. Liver energy congestion syndrome
   (0)
   None
3. Sputum-fire syndrome (7)
   Eat a lot (2)
   Excessive perspiration (2)
   Palpitations (3)
4. Liver-kidneys yin deficiency
   syndrome (3)
   Fatigue (3)
5. Deficiency fire syndrome (4)
   Becoming angry easily (2)
   Excessive perspiration (2)
6. Simultaneous deficiency of yin
   and yang syndrome (6)
   Excessive perspiration (1)
   Fatigue (3)
   Palpitations (2)

Thus, the diagnosis is 3. Sputum-
fire syndrome, with the highest score
of 7.

2
TREATMENT OF COMPLAINTS

HEADACHE

1. Wind-cold syndrome ( )

Symptoms:
Absence of perspiration (1)
Breathing through the nose (1)
Clear discharge from nose (1)
Cough (1)
Cough with heavy, unclear sounds
  and clear sputum (1)
Diarrhea (1)
Dislike of cold (1)
Dizziness (1)
Facial paralysis (1)
Fever (1)
Headache with stiff neck (2)*
Headache with dizziness (1)
Hoarseness at the beginning of
  illness (1)
Loss of voice (1)
Nosebleed (1)
Pain in the body shifting around with
  no fixed region (1)
Pain in the joints (1)
Stuffed nose (1)
Vomiting (1)
Treatment principle: to disperse
  wind and cold and stop headache
Treatment formula: *Chuan-Xiong-
  Cha-Tiao-San*
Food cures: peppermint (including
  oil), spearmint, sweet basil,
cayenne pepper, fennel, fresh
ginger, mustard seed, star anise,
prickly ash leaf, fresh ginger,
green onion, chicken egg, and
red-beet sugar

2. Wind-heat syndrome ( )

Symptoms:
Asthma (1)
Cough (1)
Coughing out blood (1)
Dizziness (1)
Headache with swelling of the head
  (3)*
Headache with dizziness (1)
Intolerance of light in eyes with
  swelling and dislike of wind (1)
Muddy discharge from nose (1)
Nosebleed (1)
Pain in the eyes (1)
Pain in the throat (1)
Red eyes (1)
Ringing in ears and deafness (1)
Tenesmus (1)
Thirst (1)
Toothache (1)
Yellow urine (1)
Yellowish discharge from the nose (1)
Treatment principle: to disperse
  wind and heat and stop pain
Treatment formula: *Sang-Ju-Yin*

Food cures: banana, bitter endive, black fungus, salt, spinach, strawberry, bamboo shoot, cucumber, Job's-tears, liver, leaf beet, mung bean, peppermint, purslane, lily flower, salt, and cattail

3. Wind-dampness syndrome ( )

Symptoms:
Chronic backache (1)
Diarrhea (1)
Eczema (1)
Edema (1)
Fever that becomes more severe in the afternoon (1)
German measles (1)
Headache with heavy or tight sensations in the head (3)*
Heavy sensations in the body (6)*
Itchy sores (1)
Light swelling (1)
Pain in all the joints (1)
Pain shifting around with no fixed region (1)
Scant urine (1)
Treatment principle: to drive out wind, overcome dampness, and relieve pain
Treatment formula: Qiang-Huo-Sheng-Shi-Tang
Food cures: Job's-tears, orange peel, peppermint, spearmint, sweet basil, celery, coconut meat, green onion, jellyfish skin, prickly ash, rice, adzuki bean, rosin, and tangerine

4. Liver yang upsurging syndrome ( )

Symptoms:
Bitter taste in the mouth (1)
Dizziness (1)
Feeling insecure while asleep (1)
Headache (1)
Headache in women (1)
Headache on the side of the head (5)*
Headache with dizziness (1)
Headache with severe pain and swelling (1)
Heavy sensations in head and light sensations in feet (1)
Misty vision (1)
Numbness (1)
Numbness of fingers (1)
Pain and swelling in the ribs (1)
Pain in the ribs (1)
Red complexion (1)
Ringing in ears and deafness (1)
Treatment principle: to calm the liver and oppress the yang and to stop the wind and relieve pain
Treatment formula: Zhen-Gan-Xi-Feng-Tang
Food cures: chicken egg yolk, cheese, kidney bean, abalone, cuttlefish, duck, duck egg, white fungus, oyster, pork, royal jelly, and celery

5. Dampness-sputum syndrome ( )

Symptoms:
Cough (1)
Discharge of sputum that can be coughed out easily (1)
Discharge of white, watery sputum (1)
Dizziness (1)
Excessive whitish vaginal discharge (1)
Frequent coughs during pregnancy that are prolonged and cause motion of fetus (1)
Headache with dizziness (3)*
Hiccups (1)
Pain in the chest (1)

49

Panting (1)
Prolonged dizziness (1)
Sleep a lot (1)
Sleeplessness (1)
Suppression of menses (1)
Vomiting (1)
White, sliding sputum that can be cleared from throat easily (1)
Whitish vaginal discharge (1)
Women susceptible to morning sickness during pregnancy (1)

Treatment principle: to transform sputum and mobilize the spleen and to relieve pain

Treatment formula: *Ban-Xia-Xie-Xin-Tang*

Food cures: peppermint, spearmint, sweet basil, celery, coconut meat, green onion, asparagus, bamboo shoot, date, leaf or brown mustard, mustard seed, black and white pepper, fresh ginger, and crown daisy

6. Energy deficiency syndrome ( )

Symptoms:
Discharge of sticky, muddy stools or diarrhea (1)
Dizziness (1)
Edema in socket of eyeball (1)
Fatigued eyes and spirits (1)
Feeble breath with a short and feeble voice (1)
Headache (severe) that occurs with fatigue after labor (2)*
Headache at intervals (2)*
Headache in the morning (2)*
Lack of appetite (1)
Pain may be relieved by massage (3)*
Perspiration on hands and feet (1)
Prolonged headache (2)*
Swallowing difficulty (1)
Tips of four limbs slightly cold (1)
Underweight with dry skin (1)

Treatment principle: to tone energy and elevate the yang and to nourish body energy

Treatment formula: *Bu-Zhong-Yi-Qi-Tang*

Food cures: grape, longan nuts, maltose, mandarin fish, Irish potato, sweet rice, apple cucumber, bog bean, gold carp, carrot, chestnut, ham, horse bean, hyacinth bean, Job's-tears, royal jelly, string bean, whitefish, yam, red and black date, mutton, squash, and rock sugar

7. Blood deficiency syndrome ( )

Symptoms:
Constipation (1)
Dizziness (1)
Dry and cracked lips and mouth (1)
Dry sensations in the mouth (1)
Fatigue (1)
Fever (1)
Headache as if being pulled by a string (3)*
Headache in the afternoon (3)*
Headache with dizziness (3)*
Lying down with an inability to sit up, which will cause dizziness (1)
Night sweats (1)
Sleeplessness (1)
Underweight with dry skin (1)
White complexion (1)

Treatment principle: to nourish the blood, soften up the liver, and stop the pain

Treatment formula: *Si-Wu-Tang*

Food cures: abalone, asparagus, cuttlefish, chicken egg, duck egg, white fungus, beef liver, grape, mandarin fish, oyster, milk, beef, cherry, blood clam, and longan nuts

8. Kidneys energy deficiency syndrome ( )

Symptoms:
Anuria (complete suppression of urination) (1)
Asthma (1)
Deafness (1)
Dizziness (1)
Fatigue (1)
Headache as if a ball were inside the head (5)*
Headache with ringing inside the head (5)*
Impotence (1)
Lumbago (1)
Prolonged dizziness (1)
Ringing in ears (1)
Seminal emission (1)
Treatment principle: to improve the essence of the kidneys and stop pain
Treatment formula: Shen-Qi-Wan
Food cures: milk, millet, stamens, sword bean, wheat, black sesame seed, beef kidney, chestnut, chicken liver, lobster, perch, pork kidney, raspberry, sea cucumber, string bean, and walnut

9. Blood coagulations syndrome ( )

Symptoms:
Abdominal pain (2)
Chest pain (?)
Coughing out blood (1)
Headache caused by external injuries (4)*
Headache with fixed pain (3)*
Lumbago (2)
Pain in the upper abdomen or the ribs (2)
Prickling pain in the head (1)
Stomachache (2)
Vomiting of blood (1)

Treatment principle: to activate the blood and remove coagulations
Treatment formula: Tao-Hong-Si-Wu-Tang
Food cures: ambergris, brown sugar, chestnut, eggplant, peach, black soybean, sturgeon, sweet basil, crab, distillers' grains, papaya, and saffron

DIZZINESS

1. Liver-fire upsurging syndrome ( )

Symptoms:
Acute dizziness (2)*
Bleeding from stomach (1)
Congested chest (1)
Deafness (1)
Depressed and hot (1)
Dim eyes (1)
Dry sensations in the mouth (1)
Getting angry easily (1)
Headache on both sides of the head and in the corners of the eyes (1)
Headache that is severe (3)*
Hiccups (1)
Nosebleed (1)
Red eyes (1)
Ringing in ears (1)
Sleeplessness or sleep a lot (1)
Vomiting of blood (1)
Yellowish-red urine (1)
Treatment principle: to clear the heat in the liver and nourish the yin
Treatment formula: Long-Dan-Xie-Gan-Tang
Food cures: spinach, chestnut, shepherd's purse, rye, black fungus, vinegar, abalone, asparagus, chicken egg, white fungus, pork, and royal jelly

2. Yin deficiency with yang excess syndrome (   )

Symptoms:
Coughing out blood (1)
Dizziness with ringing in the ears (5)*
Dizziness that drags on (chronic dizziness) (5)*
Excessive sex drive (1)
Hot sensations in the body (1)
Insomnia (1)
Jumpiness (1)
Night sweats (1)
Red appearance in the zygomatic region (1)
Seminal emission (1)
"Tidal" fever (1)
Underweight (1)

Treatment principle: to tone the liver and kidneys and to oppress the liver yang

Treatment formula: *Zhen-Gan-Xi-Feng-Tang*

Food cures: peppermint, green onion, banana, bamboo shoot, bitter endive, celery, bird's nest, cheese, kidney bean, abalone, asparagus, chicken egg, cuttlefish, duck, duck egg, white fungus, oyster, pork, and royal jelly

3. Simultaneous deficiency of yin and yang syndrome (   )

Symptoms:
Cold limbs and cold sensations in the body (1)
Dizziness with ringing in the ears (6)*
Dizziness that worsens with fatigue (5)*
Fatigue (1)
Low energy (1)
Palpitations (1)
Perspiration with hot sensations in the body easily triggered by physical activities (1)
Poor spirits (1)
Ringing in ears (1)
Too tired to talk (1)
Underweight (1)

Treatment principle: to tone the liver and kidneys and to warm and assist the original energy of the body

Treatment formula: *Shen-Qi-Wan*

Food cures: beef, cherry, bird's nest, butterfish, chicken, coconut meat, date, tofu, mustard seed, sweet rice, goose meat, mutton, jackfruit, squash, sweet potato, red and black date, rice, rock sugar, caraway seed, spearmint, common button mushroom, oregano, red bean, ambergris, dill seed, garlic, sweet basil, saffron, abalone, asparagus, cuttlefish, chicken egg, duck egg, white fungus, beef liver, grape, mandarin fish, oyster, milk, blood clam, and longan nut

4. Spleen-sputum syndrome (   )

Symptoms:
Abundant saliva (1)
Dizziness with heavy sensations in the head (6)*
Dizziness that causes inability to move (6)*
Overweight, but eat only a small amount of food (1)
Poor appetite (1)
Slight fullness of the stomach (1)
Suppression of menses in women (1)
Weakened limbs (1)

Treatment principle: to dry up dampness, transform sputum, and strengthen the spleen

Treatment formula: *Ban-Xia-Bai-Zhu-Tian-Ma-Tang*

Food cures: bamboo shoot, crown daisy, date, fresh ginger, leaf or brown mustard, black and white pepper, white or yellow mustard seed, asparagus, and pear

5. Simultaneous deficiency of energy and blood syndrome ( )

Symptoms:
Bleeding of various kinds with blood in light color, often seen in consumptive diseases (1)
Dizziness that worsens with movement (7)*
Fatigue (2)
Flying objects seen in front of the eyes (1)
Insomnia (2)
Low energy (1)
Low voice (1)
Numbness of limbs (1)
Pale complexion and lips (1)
Pale nails (1)
Palpitations (2)

Treatment principle: to strengthen the spleen and nourish the heart and to tone up both the energy and the blood

Treatment formula: *Gui-Pi-Tang*

Food cures: abalone, asparagus, cuttlefish, chicken egg, duck egg, white fungus, beef liver, grape, mandarin fish, oyster, milk, beef, cherry, blood clam, longan nuts, maltose, Irish potato, sweet rice, apple cucumber, bog bean, gold carp, carrot, chestnut, ham, horse bean, hyacinth bean, Job's-tears, royal jelly, string bean, whitefish, yam, red and black date, mutton, squash, and rock sugar

RINGING IN THE EARS AND DEAFNESS

1. Wind-heat syndrome ( )

Symptoms:
Cough (1)
Coughing out blood (1)
Dizziness (1)
Headache (1)
Headache with dizziness (1)
Intolerance of light in eyes with swelling and dislike of wind (1)
Muddy discharge from nose (1)
Nasal congestion (2)*
Nosebleed (1)
Pain in the eyes (1)
Pain in the throat (1)
Red eyes (1)
Ringing in ears and deafness all of a sudden (3)*
Thirst (1)
Toothache (1)
Yellow urine (1)
Yellowish discharge from the nose (1)

Treatment principle: to clear heat and disperse wind and to expand the lungs

Treatment formula: *Yin-Qiao-San* or *Cang-Er-Zi-San*

Food cures: banana, bitter endive, black fungus, salt, spinach, strawberry, bamboo shoot, cucumber, Job's-tears, laver, leaf beet, mung bean, peppermint, purslane, spearmint, sweet basil, celery, coconut meat, and green onion

2. Hot liver syndrome ( )

Symptoms:
Bitter taste in the mouth (1)
Deafness (1)
Dry throat (1)
Head swelling (1)

Haematuria (discharge of urine containing blood) (1)
Loud ringing in ears (6)*
Morning sickness (1)
Pain in the ribs (1)
Partial suppression of lochia (1)
Pink eyes with swelling (1)
Psychological depression (1)
Sour taste in the mouth (1)
Spasms (1)
Twitching (1)
Vaginal discharge with fishy and foul odors (1)
Treatment principle: to clear heat and sedate fire
Treatment formula: *Long-Dan-Xie-Gan-Tang*
Food cures: cow's gallbladder, banana, bitter endive, black fungus, salt, spinach, strawberry, bamboo shoot, cucumber, Job's-tears, leaf beet, mung bean, peppermint, and purslane

3. Dampness-sputum syndrome ( )

Symptoms:
Cough (2)
Discharge of sputum that can be coughed out easily (1)
Discharge of white, watery sputum (1)
Dizziness (1)
Excessive whitish vaginal discharge (1)
Frequent coughs during pregnancy that are prolonged and cause motion of fetus (1)
Headache (1)
Hiccups (1)
Pain in the chest (1)
Panting (2)
Prolonged dizziness (1)
Ringing in ears with dizziness (2)*

Ringing in ears that comes and goes with varying degrees of volume (2)*
Sleep a lot (1)
Sleeplessness (1)
Vomiting (1)
White, sliding sputum that can be cleared from throat easily (1)
Treatment principle: to transform sputum and clear fire and to harmonize the stomach
Treatment formula: *Wen-Dan-Tang* or *Ban-Xia-Bai-Zhu-Tian-Ma-Tang*
Food cures: peppermint, spearmint, sweet basil, celery, coconut meat, green onion, asparagus, bamboo shoot, date, leaf or brown mustard, mustard seed, black and white pepper, fresh ginger, and crown daisy

4. Kidneys deficiency syndrome ( )

Symptoms:
Chronic backache (1)
Deafness (2)
Diarrhea (2)
Frequent miscarriage (1)
Hair falling out easily (2)
Large quantities of urine with no thirst or drink (1)
Love of lying down with desire to sleep (2)
Pain (falling) in the lower abdomen with desire for massage (1)
Ringing in ears and deafness (2)
Ringing in ears like the sound of a cicada that goes on and on (2)
Toothache (2)
Urinary disorders (2)
Treatment principle: to water yin and suppress yang and to tone the kidneys
Treatment formula: *Er-Long-Zuo-Ci-Wan* or *Da-Bu-Yin-Wan*

Food cures: abalone, asparagus, chicken egg, white fungus, black sesame seed, beef kidney, chestnut, chicken liver, lobster, pork kidney, raspberry, scallop, sea cucumber, shrimp, string bean, and walnut

LOSS OF VOICE

1. Wind-cold syndrome (   )

Symptoms:
Absence of perspiration in hot weather (1)
Asthma (1)
Breathing through the nose (1)
Clear discharge from nose (1)
Cough (1)
Cough with heavy, unclear sounds and clear sputum (1)
Diarrhea (1)
Dislike of cold (1)
Dizziness (1)
Headache (1)
Headache with dizziness (1)
Hoarseness at the beginning of illness (1)
Loss of voice that occurs all of a sudden (3)*
Nosebleed (1)
Pain in the body shifting around with no fixed region (1)
Stuffed nose (1)
Vomiting (1)
Treatment principle: to disperse wind and cold and to expand the lungs
Treatment formula: *Xing-Su-San*
Food cures: peppermint (including oil), spearmint, sweet basil, cayenne pepper, fennel, fresh ginger, mustard seed, star anise, and prickly ash leaf

2. Hot sputum syndrome (   )

Symptoms:
Asthma (1)
Coma (1)
Cough (1)
Discharge of hard, yellow sputum in lumps (1)
Discharge of sticky, turbid, and thin stools (2)
Discharge of yellow, sticky sputum in lumps (2)
Insanity (1)
Insomnia (1)
Loss of voice with heavy, unclear voice (7)*
Stools with extremely bad smell (1)
Vomiting (1)
Wheezing (3)
Treatment principle: to clear heat in the lungs and transform sputum
Treatment formula: *Er-Mu-San* or *Sang-Ju-Yin*
Food cures: banana, bitter endive, black fungus, salt, spinach, strawberry, bamboo shoot, cucumber, Job's-tears, laver, leaf beet, mung bean, peppermint, purslane, salt, cattail, agar, radish, bamboo shoot, crown daisy, date, fresh ginger, leaf or brown mustard, black and white pepper, white or yellow mustard seed, asparagus, and pear

3. Lungs-dryness syndrome (   )

Symptoms:
Coughing out blood (2)
Dry cough (2)
Dry cough without sputum or coughing out slightly sticky fluids (1)
Dry nose (1)
Dry throat (1)
Dryness in mouth and nose (1)
Flaccidity syndrome (2)
Loss of voice with hoarseness at the beginning, gradually becoming a

complete loss of voice that drags
on and on (4)*
Morbid hunger (2)
Thirst (1)
Nosebleed (2)
Pain in the throat (1)
Presence of sputum that can't be
coughed out easily (1)
Tickle in the throat (1)
Treatment principle: to clear heat
and moisten dryness of the lungs
Treatment formula: *Yang-Yin-Qing-Fei-Yin*
Food cures: almond, apple, apricot,
asparagus, white fungus, licorice,
loquat, peanut, pear peel, rock
sugar, and tangerine

4. Insufficient kidneys yin syndrome ( )

Symptoms:
Dizziness (2)
Forgetfulness (2)
Insomnia (2)
Loss of voice with hoarseness at the
beginning, gradually becoming a
complete loss of voice that drags
on and on (4)*
Physical weakness (2)
Ringing in ears (2)
Seminal emission (2)
Sore loins (2)
Teeth as dry as withered bones (2)
Treatment principle: to water the
yin, bring down fire, and
strengthen the lungs
Treatment formula: *Mai-Wei-Di-Huang-Wan*
Food cures: abalone, asparagus,
chicken egg, cuttlefish, duck, duck
egg, white fungus, oyster, pork,
royal jelly, chestnut, chicken liver,
and pork kidneys

COUGH

1. Wind-cold syndrome ( )

Symptoms:
Breathing through the nose (1)
Clear discharge from nose (1)
Cough (1)
Cough with heavy, unclear sounds
and clear sputum (3)*
Diarrhea (1)
Dislike of cold (1)
Dizziness (1)
Facial paralysis (1)
Headache (1)
Headache with dizziness (1)
Hoarseness at the beginning of
illness (1)
Loss of voice (1)
Nosebleed (1)
Pain in the body shifting around with
no fixed region (3)*
Stuffed nose (1)
Vomiting (1)
Treatment principle: to disperse
wind and cold and to expand the
lungs and stop cough
Treatment formula: *Xing-Su-San*
Food cures: peppermint (including
oil), spearmint, sweet basil,
cayenne pepper, fennel, fresh
ginger, mustard seed, star anise,
and prickly ash leaf

2. Wind-heat syndrome ( )

Symptoms:
Coughing out sticky sputum (3)*
Coughing out blood (1)
Dizziness (1)
Fever in children (1)
German measles (1)
Headache (1)
Headache with dizziness (1)
Intolerance of light in eyes with
swelling and dislike of wind (1)
Muddy discharge from nose (1)

Nosebleed (1)
Pain in the eyes (1)
Pain in the throat (1)
Red eyes (1)
Ringing in ears and deafness (1)
Tenesmus (1)
Thirst (1)
Toothache (1)
Yellow urine (1)
Yellowish discharge from the nose (1)
Treatment principle: to disperse wind and heat and to expand the lungs and stop cough
Treatment formula: *Sang-Ju-Yin*
Food cures: banana, bitter endive, black fungus, salt, spinach, strawberry, bamboo shoot, cucumber, Job's-tears, laver, leaf beet, mung bean, peppermint, purslane, spearmint, sweet basil, celery, coconut meat, and green onion

3. Dryness-heat syndrome ( )

Symptoms:
Constipation (3)
Cough with no sputum (4)*
Cough with a little sputum that is difficult to cough out (4)*
Diabetes mellitus (3)
Dry nose or dry throat (3)
Thirst (3)
Treatment principle: to clear heat, moisten dryness, produce fluids, and regulate the lungs
Treatment formula: *Sang-Xing-Tang* or *Qing-Zao-Jiu-Fei-Tang*
Food cures: asparagus, soya milk, bird's nest, cattail, chicken egg, honey, maltose, milk, pear, sesame oil, yellow soybean, banana, bitter endive, black fungus, salt, spinach, strawberry, bamboo shoot, cucumber, Job's-tears, laver, leaf beet, mung bean, peppermint, and purslane

4. Dampness-sputum syndrome ( )

Symptoms:
Cough that stops after sputum is cleared (4)*
Discharge of abundant sputum that can be coughed out easily (3)*
Discharge of white, watery sputum (1)
Dizziness (1)
Frequent coughs during pregnancy that are prolonged and cause motion of fetus (1)
Headache (1)
Hiccups (1)
Pain in the chest (1)
Panting (2)
Prolonged dizziness (1)
Sleep a lot (1)
Sleeplessness (1)
Vomiting (2)
White, sliding sputum that can be cleared from throat easily (1)
Treatment principle: to strengthen the spleen and dry up dampness and to transform sputum and regulate the lungs
Treatment formula: *Er-Chen-Tang*
Food cures: adzuki bean, ambergris, barley, common carp, cucumber, mung bean, seaweed, shepherd's purse, star fruit, bamboo shoot, crown daisy, date, fresh ginger, leaf or brown mustard, black and white pepper, white or yellow mustard seed, asparagus, and pear

5. Liver-fire upsurging syndrome ( )

Symptoms:
Acute dizziness (1)
Bleeding from stomach (2)
Cough with a sensation of something moving upward to the throat (3)*

Depressed and hot (1)
Dizziness (1)
Getting angry easily (1)
Headache on both sides of the head
and in the corners of the eyes (1)
Headache that is severe (2)
Insanity (2)
Nosebleed (1)
Red eyes (1)
Reddish-yellow urine (1)
Ringing in ears (2)
Sleeplessness or sleep a lot (1)
Treatment principle: to calm the
liver and sedate fire and to clear
the lungs and stop cough
Treatment formula: *Ke-Xue-Fang*
Food cures: spinach, chestnut,
shepherd's purse, rye, black
fungus, vinegar, abalone,
asparagus, chicken egg, white
fungus, pork, and royal jelly

6. Yin deficiency syndrome
( )

Symptoms:
Bleeding from gums (1)
Constipation (1)
Dizziness (2)
Dry and scant stools (1)
Dry cough or dry throat with little
sputum (3)*
Dry sensations in the mouth (1)
Fatigue (2)
Headache in the afternoon (1)
Light "tidal" fever that attacks in the
afternoon (1)
Night sweats (1)
Nosebleed (1)
Palms of hands and soles of feet are
both hot (1)
Sleeplessness (1)
Swallowing difficulty (1)
Toothache (1)
Underweight (1)

Treatment principle: to water the
yin and clear fire and to moisten
the lungs
Treatment formula: *Bai-He-Gu-Jin-
Tang*
Food cures: bird's nest, cheese,
kidney bean, abalone, asparagus,
chicken egg, cuttlefish, duck, duck
egg, white fungus, oyster, pork,
and royal jelly

PALPITATIONS

1. Simultaneous deficiency of energy and blood syndrome ( )

Symptoms:
Bleeding of various kinds with blood
in light color, often seen in
consumptive diseases (1)
Dizziness (3)
Fatigue (3)
Flying objects seen in front of the
eyes (1)
Insomnia (3)
Low energy (1)
Low voice (1)
Numbness of limbs (1)
Pale complexion and lips (1)
Pale nails (1)
Palpitations with insecure feeling (4)*
Treatment principle: to tone the
blood and strengthen energy and
to nourish the heart and secure
the spirits
Treatment formula: *Gui-Pi-Tang*
Food cures: abalone, asparagus,
cuttlefish, chicken egg, duck egg,
white fungus, beef liver, grape,
mandarin fish, oyster, milk, beef,
cherry, blood clam, longan nuts,
maltose, Irish potato, sweet rice,
apple cucumber, bog bean, gold
carp, carrot, chestnut, ham, horse
bean, hyacinth bean, Job's-tears,

royal jelly, string bean, whitefish, yam, red and black date, mutton, squash, and rock sugar

2. Deficiency fire syndrome ( )

Symptoms:
Coughing out blood (1)
Dry cough without sputum or coughing out slightly sticky fluids (1)
Dry sensations in the mouth (1)
Dry throat (1)
Feeling miserable with palpitations (4)*
Forgetfulness (1)
Hot sensations in body (1)
Illness attacks slowly but with a longer duration (chronic illness) (1)
Night sweats (2)
Pain in the throat (1)
Ringing in ears (1)
Seminal emission with dreams (1)
Sleeplessness (1)
Sore loins (1)
Sputum with blood (1)
Toothache (1)
Treatment principle: to water the yin and bring down the fire and to strengthen the kidneys and secure the heart
Treatment formula: Bu-Xin-Dan
Food cures: banana, bitter endive, black fungus, salt, spinach, strawberry, bamboo shoot, cucumber, Job's-tears, liver, leaf beet, mung bean, peppermint, purslane, lily flower, salt, cattail, chicken egg, duck egg, asparagus, royal jelly, pork, and oyster

3. Kidneys-water attacking the heart syndrome ( )

Symptoms:
Congested chest with abdominal swelling (1)

Cough (1)
Dizziness (5)*
Edema (3)
Fingers and lips in blue-purple color (1)
Inability to lie on back (1)
Nervousness (1)
Palpitations with a sensation of fullness below the heart (5)*
Shortness of breath (3)
Treatment principle: to warm the heart and tone the energy and to promote water flow
Treatment formula: Ling-Gui-Zhu-Gan-Tang
Food cures: dried ginger, water spinach, cinnamon, longan nut, wheat, kidney, lobster, sardine, shrimp, sparrow, clove, dill seed, fennel, pistachio nut, sparrow egg, crab apple, raspberry, and walnut

4. Heart deficiency syndrome ( )

Symptoms:
Automatic perspiration not due to hot weather or labor (1)
Deafness (1)
Feeling miserable with love of darkness and dislike of light (1)
Forgetfulness (2)
Getting scared easily (2)
Love of lying down with desire for sleep (1)
Many dreams (2)
Muscular tightening (1)
Nervousness (1)
Night sweats (1)
Palpitations with nervousness (5)*
Sleeplessness (1)
Worry a lot (1)
Treatment principle: to calm the heart and secure the spirits and to tone the heart and nourish the blood

Treatment formula: *Tian-Wang-Bu-Xin-Dan*

Food cures: soya milk, goose meat, milk, royal jelly, grape, longan nuts, mandarin fish, maltose, and Irish potato

INSOMNIA

1. Heart-spleen deficiency syndrome ( )

Symptoms:
Abdominal swelling (1)
Discharge of watery, thin stools (1)
Eating very little (1)
Fatigue (2)
Forgetfulness (2)
Impotence (1)
Many dreams (1)
Nervous spirits (1)
Nervousness (2)
Night sweats (1)
Palpitations (2)
Poor appetite (3)*
Shortness of breath (1)
Sleeplessness and wake up easily (1)
Withering and yellowish complexion (1)

Treatment principle: to tone the heart and the spleen and to secure the heart and calm the spirits

Treatment formula: *Gui-Pi-Tang* or *Yang-Xin-Tang*

Food cures: beef liver, chicken egg, cuttlefish, oyster, pork liver, sea cucumber, water spinach, longan nut, mandarin fish, apple cucumber, chestnut, horse bean, Job's-tears, Irish potato, rice, royal jelly, and yam

2. Heart-kidneys unable to communicate with each other syndrome ( )

Symptoms:
Deafness (1)
Dizziness (1)
Face becomes red when fatigued or working hard (1)
Feeling miserable (1)
Forgetfulness (2)
Light but periodic fever not unlike the tide (1)
Nervousness (2)
Night sweats (1)
Palpitations (2)
Ringing in ears (1)
Seminal emission (2)
Sleeplessness due to stress or depression (3)*
Sleeplessness with forgetfulness (1)

Treatment principle: to water yin and clear fire and to promote communication between the heart and the kidneys

Treatment formula: *Huang-Lian-E-Jiao-Tang*

Food cures: asparagus, abalone, chicken egg, white fungus, bog bean, wheat, banana, bamboo shoot, bitter endive, oyster, royal jelly, and pork

3. Heart-gallbladder deficiency syndrome ( )

Symptoms:
Bitter taste in the mouth (3)
Depressed with a desire to vomit (3)
Feeling miserable with love of darkness and dislike of light (2)
Insomnia due to nervousness (5)*
Scared by events easily (2)
Wake up at night easily due to shock (5)*

Treatment principle: to strengthen energy, overcome nervousness, and secure the spirits

Treatment formula: *An-Shen-Ding-Zhi-Wan*

Food cures: corn silk, cow's gallbladder, air bladder of shark, water spinach, abalone, asparagus, dried ginger, and cinnamon

4. Sputum-fire syndrome (   )

Symptoms:
Difficult defecation or urination (2)
Hungry with no appetite (2)
Insanity (3)
Ringing in ears and deafness (3)
Sleeplessness due to congested chest (10)*
Treatment principle: to transform sputum and harmonize the middle region
Treatment formula: Wen-Dan-Tang
Food cures: salt, cattail, agar, radish, bamboo shoot, crown daisy, date, fresh ginger, leaf or brown mustard, black and white pepper, white or yellow mustard seed, asparagus, and pear

5. Indigestion syndrome (   )

Symptoms:
Abdominal pain (1)
Abdominal pain with a desire for massage (1)
Abdominal pain with an aversion to massage (1)
Abdominal distension (5)*
Belching of bad breath after meals (1)
Chest and diaphragm congestion and discomfort (1)
Diarrhea and constipation (1)
Hot sensations in the middle of palms (1)
Indigestion (1)
Lack of appetite (1)
Love of hot drink, but drink very little (1)
Nausea (1)
Pain in inner part of stomach with swelling and feeling of fullness (1)
Stomachache (1)

Stools with an extremely bad smell (1)
Vomiting of clear water (1)
Treatment principle: to promote digestion and harmonize the middle region
Treatment formula: Bao-He-Wan
Food cures: asafoetida, buckwheat, castor bean, jellyfish, peach, radish, water chestnut, cardamon seed, cayenne pepper, coriander, grapefruit, jackfruit, malt, sweet basil, tea, and tomato

TICS

1. Wind syndrome (   )

Symptoms:
Diarrhea containing undigested food (1)
Discharge of watery, thin stools (1)
Dislike of wind (1)
Excessive perspiration (1)
Headache accompanied by fear of wind (1)
Headache with heavy sensations in the head (1)
Illness (acute) attacking all of a sudden (1)
Itch (1)
Itchy skin that becomes almost intolerable (1)
Light cough (1)
Nasal discharge (1)
Numbness in the skin of the face (1)
Pain in all the joints that attacks suddenly (1)
Pain in the joints that shifts from one joint to another (1)
Shaking of four limbs and body (1)
Sneezing (1)
Stiffness of muscles (1)
Stuffed nose with heavy voice (1)
Tickle in the throat (1)
Wry mouth (1)

Treatment principle: to expel wind and transform sputum and to relieve spasms and overcome convulsions

Treatment formula: *Wu-Hu-Zhui-Feng-San*

Food cures: peppermint, spearmint, sweet basil, celery, coconut meat, and green onion

2. Extreme heat generating wind syndrome ( )

Symptoms:
Convulsions (2)
Fainting (2)
Feeling troubled, quick-tempered, and insecure (2)
High fever (6)
Muscular tightening (2)
Neck stiffness (2)
Twitching or spasms of four limbs (2)
Wry and shivering tongue (2)

Treatment principle: to clear heat and stop convulsions

Treatment formula: *An-Gong-Niu-Huang-Wan*

Food cures: peppermint, spearmint, sweet basil, celery, coconut meat, green onion, chicken egg, bitter endive, camellia, cattail, black fungus, salt, spinach, strawberry, banana, bamboo shoot, crab, and water clam

3. Blood deficiency generating wind syndrome ( )

Symptoms:
Dizziness (2)
Fainting (2)
Muscular (spasmodic) contractions (2)
Muscular tightening (2)
Numbness of hands and feet (2)
Pain in the upper abdomen (2)
Ringing in ears (2)
Shaking of hands and feet (2)
Spots in front of the eyes (2)
Twitching (2)

Treatment principle: to strengthen the liver and the kidneys and to stop convulsions

Treatment formula: *Da-Ding-Feng-Zhu*

Food cures: egg, mulberry, abalone, liver, cuttlefish, grape, milk, and brown sugar

4. Simultaneous deficiency of energy and blood syndrome ( )

Symptoms:
Bleeding of various kinds with blood in light color, often seen in consumptive diseases (1)
Dizziness (3)
Fatigue (2)
Flying objects seen in front of the eyes (1)
Insomnia (2)
Low energy (1)
Low voice (1)
Numbness of limbs (5)*
Pale complexion and lips (1)
Pale nails (1)
Palpitations (2)

Treatment principle: to tone energy in order to produce the blood and to nourish the blood in order to nourish the tendons

Treatment formula: *Ba-Zhen-Tang*

Food cures: abalone, asparagus, cuttlefish, chicken egg, duck egg, white fungus, beef liver, grape, mandarin fish, oyster, milk, beef, cherry, blood clam, longan nuts, maltose, Irish potato, sweet rice, apple cucumber, bog bean, gold carp, carrot, chestnut, ham, horse bean, hyacinth bean, Job's-tears, royal jelly, string bean, whitefish, yam, red and black date, mutton, squash, and rock sugar

5. Heart-gallbladder deficiency syndrome ( )

Symptoms:
Bitter taste in the mouth (4)
Depressed with a desire to vomit (2)
Feeling miserable with love of darkness and dislike of light (2)
Insomnia (2)
Scared by events easily (2)
Sleeplessness (2)
Trembling that is often triggered by nervousness (6)*
Treatment principle: to tone the energy of the heart and to overcome nervousness and secure the spirits
Treatment formula: Gan-Mai-Da-Zao-Tang
Food cures: corn silk, cow's gallbladder, air bladder of shark, water spinach, abalone, asparagus, dried ginger, and cinnamon

COUGHING OUT BLOOD

1. Wind-dryness syndrome ( )

Symptoms:
Blood in sputum (5)*
Chest pain (1)
Coughing with scant sputum (1)
Dry nose (1)
Dry skin with wrinkles (1)
Dry throat (1)
Dry, withered fingernails (1)
Fever (1)
Headache (1)
Itch in the throat (4)*
No perspiration (1)
Pain in the upper abdomen (1)

Symptoms attack or worsen in autumn or in a dry climate (1)
Thirst (1)
Treatment principle: to disperse wind and heat and to lubricate the lungs
Treatment formula: Sang-Xing-Tang or Si-Sheng-Wan
Food cures: peppermint, spearmint, sweet basil, celery, coconut meat, green onion, asparagus, egg, honey, pear, sesame oil, yellow soybean, spinach, and tofu

2. Liver-fire upsurging syndrome ( )

Symptoms:
Acute dizziness (1)
Bleeding from stomach (1)
Coughing out sputum with blood in it or coughing out fresh blood (3)*
Deafness (1)
Dim vision (1)
Dizziness (1)
Dry sensations in the mouth (1)
Getting angry easily (1)
Headache on both sides of the head and in the corners of the eyes (1)
Headache that is severe (2)
Nosebleed (1)
Pain (falling) in the lower abdomen with desire for massage (1)
Pain in the upper abdomen (1)
Pink eyes with swelling (1)
Reddish-yellow urine (1)
Red eyes (1)
Ringing in ears (1)
Sleeplessness or sleep a lot (1)
Treatment principle: to sedate the liver, lubricate the lungs, and stop bleeding
Treatment formula: Ke-Xue-Fang
Food cures: spinach, chestnut, shepherd's purse, rye, black fungus, vinegar, abalone,

asparagus, chicken egg, white fungus, pork, and royal jelly

3. Yin deficiency syndrome ( )

Symptoms:
Bleeding from gums (1)
Constipation (1)
Coughing out abundant blood in light color (3)*
Dizziness (2)
Dry and scant stools (1)
Dry sensations in the mouth or the throat (1)
Fatigue (2)
Headache in the afternoon (1)
Night sweats (1)
Pain in the throat, also red and swollen (1)
Palms of hands and soles of feet are both hot (1)
Short and reddish streams of urine (1)
Sleeplessness (1)
Swallowing difficulty (1)
Toothache (1)
Underweight (1)
Treatment principle: to water the yin, clear heat, lubricate dryness, and stop bleeding
Treatment formula: *Bai-He-Gu-Jin-Tang*
Food cures: bird's nest, cheese, kidney bean, abalone, asparagus, chicken egg, cuttlefish, duck, duck egg, white fungus, oyster, pork, and royal jelly

VOMITING OF BLOOD

1. Hot stomach syndrome ( )

Symptoms:
Bad breath (1)
Bleeding from gums (1)
Foul breath from the mouth (1)

Getting hungry easily (1)
Gums swelling (1)
Hiccups (1)
Morning sickness (1)
Nosebleed (1)
Pain in the gums with swelling (2)
Pain in the throat (1)
Perspiring on the head (1)
Stomachache (2)
Thirst and craving for cold (1)
Vomiting of fresh blood or blood mixed with foods (3)*
Vomiting right after eating (1)
Vomiting with stomach discomfort as if hungry, empty, or hot (1)
Treatment principle: to clear the heat in the stomach, sedate fire, cool the blood, and stop bleeding
Treatment formula: *Xie-Xin-Tang*
Food cures: salt, lily flower, bitter endive, camellia, cattail, black fungus, spinach, strawberry, banana, cucumber, and licorice

2. Stomach-fire syndrome ( )

Symptoms:
Bitter taste in the mouth (1)
Bleeding from gums (1)
Constipation (1)
Depressed, quick-tempered, and insecure (1)
Dry sensations in the mouth (1)
Eating a lot and still feeling hungry (1)
Fever (1)
Headache (1)
Hiccups (1)
Hungry with good appetite, and eat a lot but still underweight (1)
Nosebleed (1)
Pain in the gums with swelling (1)
Pain in the throat, also red and swollen (1)
Screaming during sleep in children (1)

Toothache (1)

Vomiting of blood that occurs all of a sudden and in huge amounts (2)*

Vomiting of red or dark blood (2)*

Vomiting right after eating (1)

Treatment principle: to clear the heat in the liver, cool the blood, and stop bleeding

Treatment formula: *Yu-Nü-Jian*

Food cures: areca nuts, buckwheat, common carp, banana, bitter endive, black fungus, salt, spinach, strawberry, bamboo shoot, cucumber, Job's-tears, liver, leaf beet, mung bean, peppermint, purslane, lily flower, salt, and cattail

3. Spleen unable to govern the blood syndrome ( )

Symptoms:

Blood in urine (2)

Discharge of blood from anus (2)

Discharge of sticky, muddy stools or diarrhea (1)

Dizziness (1)

Mentally fatigued (1)

Nosebleed (2)

Palpitations (1)

Poor appetite (2)

Pure-white complexion (2)

Shortness of breath (1)

Stomach and abdomen swelling and fullness (1)

Vomiting of dark- and light-colored blood that recurs frequently (3)*

Withering and yellowish complexion (1)

Treatment principle: to tone the energy and the blood and to constrict the blood and stop bleeding

Treatment formula: *Huang-Tu-Tang*

Food cures: chicken, grape, longan nuts, maltose, mandarin fish, Irish

potato, sweet rice, apple cucumber, bog bean, gold carp, carrot, chestnut, ham, horse bean, hyacinth bean, Job's-tears, royal jelly, string bean, whitefish, yam, red and black date, mutton, squash, rock sugar, and chicken egg yolk

NOSEBLEED

1. Hot lungs syndrome ( )

Symptoms:

Acute panting in high-pitched sound with rapid expiration (1)

Bitter taste in the mouth (1)

Cough with subdued and oppressed sounds (1)

Coughing out and vomiting of pus and blood with a fishy smell (1)

Coughing out yellow and sticky sputum (1)

Discharge of dry stools (1)

Dry nose (3)*

Dry sensations in the mouth (1)

Flickering of nostrils (1)

Hot sensations in the body (1)

Light but periodic fever not unlike the tide (1)

Nosebleed with fresh blood (3)*

Pain in the chest or in the throat (1)

Presence of sputum that can't be coughed out easily (1)

Psychological depression (1)

Urgent panting (1)

Treatment principle: to sedate the lungs and clear the heat in the lungs and to cool the blood and stop bleeding

Treatment formula: *Sang-Xing-Tang* or *He-Ye-Wan*

Food cures: apple, apple cucumber, apricot, white fungus, ham, jackfruit, lemon, maltose, mandarin orange, mulberry, olive, peach, pear, sweet potato, red and black date, tomato, white sugar, mung bean, and eggplant

2. Hot stomach syndrome ( )

Symptoms:
Bad breath (3)*
Bleeding from gums (1)
Dry nose (2)*
Nosebleed with blood in fresh red color (2)*
Pain in the gums with swelling (2)
Pain in the throat (1)
Perspiring on the head (1)
Stomachache (2)
Thirst and craving for cold (1)
Vomiting (2)
Vomiting of blood (2)
Vomiting right after eating (1)
Treatment principle: to clear the heat in the stomach, nourish the yin, and cool the blood and stop bleeding
Treatment formula: *Yu-Nü-Jian*
Food cures: salt, lily flower, bitter endive, camellia, cattail, black fungus, spinach, strawberry, banana, cucumber, and licorice

3. Hot liver syndrome ( )

Symptoms:
Bitter taste in the mouth (1)
Blood in urine (1)
Deafness (1)
Dry throat (1)
Head swelling or headache (3)*
Nosebleed with abundant blood in fresh red color (4)*
Pain in the upper abdomen (3)*
Partial suppression of lochia (1)
Pink eyes with swelling (1)
Psychological depression (1)
Sour taste in the mouth (1)
Spasms (1)
Twitching (1)

Vaginal discharge with fishy and foul odors (1)
Treatment principle: to calm the liver and clear the heat in the liver and to cool the blood and stop bleeding
Treatment formula: *Long-Dan-Xie-Gan-Tang*
Food cures: cow's gallbladder, banana, bitter endive, black fungus, salt, spinach, strawberry, bamboo shoot, cucumber, Job's-tears, leaf beet, mung bean, peppermint, and purslane

BLOOD IN URINE

1. Heart-fire syndrome ( )

Symptoms:
Bleeding from gums (1)
Burning sensations on urination (3)*
Cold hands and feet (1)
Discharge of blood from the mouth (1)
Dribbling after urination (1)
Feeling miserable (1)
Hot sensations in the middle of palms (1)
Morning sickness (1)
Mouth canker (1)
Not alert (1)
Pain on urination (1)
Palpitations (1)
Pulpy and decayed tongue and mouth (1)
Reddish-yellow urine (1)
Seminal emission (1)
Short streams of urine (1)
Sleeplessness (1)
Urine blood in fresh red color (1)
Treatment principle: to clear the heat in the heart and to cool the blood and stop bleeding
Treatment formula: *Xiao-Ji-Yin-Zi*
Food cures: asparagus, pear peel, banana, bitter endive, black

fungus, salt, spinach, strawberry, bamboo shoot, cucumber, Job's-tears, liver, leaf beet, mung bean, peppermint, purslane, lily flower, salt, and cattail

2. Dampness-heat flowing downward syndrome ( )

Symptoms:
Abdominal pain (1)
Burning sensations and itch in the genitals (4)*
Congested chest (1)
Diarrhea (1)
Fever that doesn't appear high (1)
Jaundice (1)
Urine blood in fresh red color (3)*
Perspiration on hands and feet (1)
Reddish and scant urine (1)
Retention of urine (1)
Short and reddish streams of urine (1)
Swollen body of the tongue (1)
Thirst (1)
Treatment principle: to clear the heat in the bladder and promote urination and to cool the blood and stop bleeding
Treatment formula: *Ba-Zheng-San*
Food cures: carp, celery, horse bean, jellyfish skin, Job's-tears, prickly ash, hyacinth bean, oregano, sweet basil, adzuki bean, bamboo shoot, soybean sprouts, rosin, banana, bitter endive, black fungus, salt, spinach, strawberry, cucumber, leaf beet, mung bean, peppermint, and purslane

3. Simultaneous deficiency of energy and blood syndrome ( )

Symptoms:
Bleeding of various kinds with blood in light color, often seen in consumptive diseases (1)

Dizziness (3)
Fatigue (3)
Flying objects seen in front of the eyes (1)
Insomnia (3)
Low energy (1)
Low voice (1)
No burning sensation on urination (1)
Numbness of limbs (1)
Pale complexion and lips (1)
Pale nails (1)
Palpitations (3)
Treatment principle: to tone the energy and the blood and to constrict the blood and stop bleeding
Treatment formula: *Gui-Pi-Tang* or *Huang-Tu-Tang*
Food cures: abalone, asparagus, cuttlefish, chicken egg, duck egg, white fungus, beef liver, grape, mandarin fish, oyster, milk, beef, cherry, blood clam, longan nuts, maltose, Irish potato, sweet rice, apple cucumber, bog bean, gold carp, carrot, chestnut, ham, horse bean, hyacinth bean, Job's-tears, royal jelly, string bean, whitefish, yam, red and black date, mutton, squash, and rock sugar

4. Kidneys deficiency syndrome ( )

Symptoms:
Asthma (1)
Chronic backache (2)
Clear, watery, and whitish vaginal discharge (1)
Deafness (2)
Diarrhea (2)
Hair falling out easily (2)
Large quantities of urine with no thirst or drink (1)
Love of lying down with desire to sleep (1)

No burning sensation on urination
(2)
Pain (falling) in the lower abdomen
with desire for massage (1)
Ringing in ears (1)
Ringing in ears and deafness (2)
Seminal emission (1)
Toothache (1)
Treatment principle: to water the
yin and strengthen the kidneys
and to constrict the blood and
stop bleeding
Treatment formula: *Liu-Wei-Di-
Huang-Wan* or *Da-Bu-Yin-Wan*
Food cures: abalone, asparagus,
chicken egg, white fungus, black
sesame seed, beef kidney,
chestnut, chicken liver, lobster,
pork kidney, raspberry, scallop,
sea cucumber, shrimp, string
bean, and walnut

BLOOD IN STOOL

1. Spleen unable to govern the blood syndrome (   )

Symptoms:
Blood in urine (1)
Bowel movements, followed by
bleeding (4)*
Discharge of blood from anus with
blood in dark color (4)*
Discharge of sticky, muddy stools or
diarrhea (1)
Dizziness (1)
Mentally fatigued (1)
Nosebleed (2)
Palpitations (1)
Poor appetite (1)
Pure-white complexion (1)
Shortness of breath (1)
Stomach and abdomen swelling and
fullness (1)
Withering and yellowish complexion
(1)

Treatment principle: to strengthen
the spleen and warm the middle
region and to constrict the blood
and stop bleeding
Treatment formula: *Gui-Pi-Tang* or
Huang-Tu-Tang
Food cures: chicken, grape, longan
nuts, maltose, mandarin fish, Irish
potato, sweet rice, apple
cucumber, bog bean, gold carp,
carrot, chestnut, ham, horse bean,
hyacinth bean, Job's-tears, royal
jelly, string bean, whitefish, yam,
red and black date, mutton,
squash, rock sugar, and chicken
egg yolk

2. Large-intestine dampness-heat syndrome (   )

Symptoms:
Abdominal pain (2)
Bleeding, following by bowel
movement (3)*
Blood in fresh-red color (4)*
Damp, glossy, and reddened anus in
children (1)
Diarrhea with stools containing pus
and blood (2)
Discharge of blood from anus (1)
Dysentery (2)
Hemorrhoids (3)
Pain in anus with swelling and
burning sensations (2)
Short and reddish streams of urine
(1)
Treatment principle: to clear the
dampness-heat in the large
intestine and to cool the blood
and stop bleeding
Treatment formula: *Chi-Xiao-Dou-
Dang-Gui-San, Huai-Hua-San*
Food cures: hyacinth bean, mackerel,
sweet basil, day lily, abalone,
adzuki bean, celery, chicken egg
white, mung bean, Job's-tears,
jellyfish, and eggplant

VOMITING

1. Cold-dampness syndrome ( )

Symptoms:
Absence of perspiration in hot weather (1)
Cold sensations in lower abdomen–genitals region (1)
Cough (1)
Coughing out sputum with a low sound (1)
Diarrhea (2)
Discharge of sputum that can be coughed out easily (1)
Dysentery (2)
Edema in the four limbs (1)
Headache (1)
Movement difficulty (1)
Nausea (4)*
Pain in the body (1)
Pain in the joints (1)
Scant and clear urine (1)
Stomachache (1)

Treatment principle: to disperse cold, dry up dampness, harmonize the stomach, and stop vomiting

Treatment formula: *Huo-Xiang-Zheng-Qi-San*

Food cures: cayenne pepper, dill seed, fennel, fresh ginger, mustard seed, prickly ash, star anise, white or yellow mustard, wine, carp, celery, horse bean, jellyfish skin, Job's-tears, hyacinth bean, oregano, sweet basil, adzuki bean, bamboo shoot, soybean sprouts, and rosin

2. Indigestion syndrome ( )

Symptoms:
Abdominal pain (1)
Abdominal pain with a desire for massage (1)
Abdominal pain with an aversion to massage (1)
Belching of bad breath after meals (3)*
Chest and diaphragm congestion and discomfort (1)
Diarrhea and constipation (1)
Diarrhea in children (1)
Hot sensations in the middle of palms (1)
Indigestion (1)
Lack of appetite (1)
Love of hot drink, but drink only a little (1)
Malaria (1)
Nausea (1)
Pain in inner part of stomach with swelling and feeling of fullness (1)
Stomachache (1)
Stools with an extremely bad smell (1)
Vomiting of clear water or rotten acid (2)*

Treatment principle: to promote digestion, harmonize the stomach, and stop vomiting

Treatment formula: *Bao-He-Wan*

Food cures: asafoetida, buckwheat, castor bean, jellyfish, peach, radish, water chestnut, cardamon seed, cayenne pepper, coriander, grapefruit, jackfruit, malt, sweet basil, tea, and tomato

3. Dampness-sputum syndrome ( )

Symptoms:
Cough (1)
Discharge of sputum that can be coughed out easily (1)
Discharge of white-watery sputum (1)
Dizziness (1)
Headache (1)
Hiccups (1)
Pain in the chest (1)
Panting (3)

Prolonged dizziness (2)
Sleep a lot (2)
Sleeplessness (2)
Vomiting of watery sputum (3)
White, sliding sputum that can be cleared from throat easily (2)
Treatment principle: to warm and transform sputum and to harmonize the stomach and stop vomiting
Treatment formula: *Xiao-Ban-Xia-Tang*
Food cures: adzuki bean, ambergris, barley, common carp, cucumber, mung bean, seaweed, shepherd's purse, star fruit, bamboo shoot, crown daisy, date, fresh ginger, leaf or brown mustard, black and white pepper, white or yellow mustard seed, asparagus, and pear

4. Stomach energy upsurging syndrome ( )

Symptoms:
Dysphagia (2)
Dry vomiting (2)
Eating in the evening and vomiting in the morning (2)
Eating in the morning and vomiting in the evening (2)
Hiccups in short sounds (2)
Nausea (2)
Upset stomach (3)
Vomiting of foods, watery sputum, or acidic and bitter water (3)*
Vomiting right after eating (2)
Treatment principle: to harmonize the stomach, regulate stomach energy, and stop vomiting
Treatment formula: *Xuan-Fu-Dai-Zhe-Tang*
Food cures: almond, areca nut, sugar beet, brake, buckwheat, common carp, cashew nut, coriander, loquat, malt, pea, black and white

pepper, radish, rice bran, and sword bean

5. Yang deficiency syndrome ( )

Symptoms:
Clear and long streams of urine (1)
Cold hands and feet (1)
Constipation (1)
Diarrhea (1)
Diminished urination (1)
Discharge of watery, thin stools (1)
Edema (1)
Fatigue with lack of power (1)
Fear of cold (1)
Fingertips often cold (1)
Frequent fear of cold both in hands and feet (1)
Frequent illness and love of sleep (1)
Head and body curled up while lying down (1)
Headache in the morning (1)
Palpitations (1)
Perspiration like cold water (1)
Scant energy and too tired to talk (1)
Sleep a lot (1)
Vomiting of clear water (1)*
Vomiting right after a full meal (1)*
Treatment principle: to warm the middle region and strengthen the spleen and to strengthen the stomach and stop vomiting
Treatment formula: *Li-Zhong-Tang* or *Wu-Zhu-Yu-Tang*
Food cures: kidneys, lobster, sardine, shrimp, star anise, and red and black date

6. Yin deficiency syndrome ( )

Symptoms:
Bleeding from gums (1)
Constipation (1)
Dizziness (2)

Dry sensations in the mouth (1)
Dry throat (1)
Dry vomiting (3)*
Fatigue (1)
Headache in the afternoon (1)
Light fever in the afternoon (1)
Night sweats (1)
Nosebleed (1)
Pain in the throat (1)
Short and reddish streams of urine (1)
Sleeplessness (1)
Swallowing difficulty (1)
Toothache (1)
Underweight (1)
Treatment principle: to water the yin and nourish the stomach and to lubricate dryness and stop vomiting
Treatment formula: *Sha-Shen-Mai-Dong-Tang*
Food cures: bird's nest, cheese, kidney bean, abalone, asparagus, chicken egg, cuttlefish, duck, duck egg, white fungus, oyster, pork, and royal jelly

HICCUPS

1. Cold syndrome ( )

Symptoms:
Constipation (1)
Coughing out and vomiting bubbles of saliva (1)
Dislike of cold or dislike of talking (1)
Dizziness with objects appearing in front of eyes (1)
Dry throat (1)
Hands and feet extremely cold (1)
Heavy and unclear voice with high-pitched and rough tone (1)
Hiccups with loud and forceful sounds (2)*
Hiccups with cold hands and feet and easily started by cold air (2)*

Love of hot drink (1)
Pain in inner part of stomach, getting better after meals (1)
Pain shifting around with no fixed region (1)
Pale complexion (1)
Plenty of saliva (1)
Severe pain in the joints (1)
Sore loins and weak legs (1)
Thinking about water but with no desire to drink it (1)
Whitish urine (1)
Treatment principle: to warm the middle region and disperse cold and to harmonize the stomach and stop hiccups
Treatment formula: *Ding-Xiang-Shi-Di-Tang*
Food cures: cayenne pepper, dill seed, fennel, fresh ginger, mustard seed, prickly ash, star anise, white or yellow mustard, and wine

2. Hot syndrome ( )

Symptoms:
Constipation or diarrhea (1)
Depressed, quick-tempered, and insecure (1)
Diminished urination (1)
Discharge of copious, yellow, sticky sputum (1)
Dry lips or dry teeth (1)
Escape of gas from the anus with noise (1)
Hiccups that make loud and short sound, with dryness and thirst (2)*
Hiccups that make quick sound and occur quite frequently (2)*
Light fever (1)
Light sensations in the body that can turn easily (1)
Limbs are warm (1)
Little saliva (1)
Love of cold or cold drink (1)

Stools with an extremely bad smell (1)

Thirst with an incessant desire to drink (1)

Throat swelling and red, producing rotten liquid (1)

Urine with an extremely bad smell (1)

Vomiting of sour, bad-smelling foods, with a love of cold drink (1)

Treatment principle: to clear the heat and sedate the fire and to harmonize the stomach and stop hiccups

Treatment formula: *Zhu-Ye-Shi-Gao-Tang*

Food cures: banana, bitter endive, black fungus, salt, spinach, strawberry, bamboo shoot, cucumber, Job's-tears, laver, leaf beet, mung bean, peppermint, and purslane

3. Indigestion syndrome ( )

Symptoms:
Abdominal pain (1)

Abdominal pain with a desire for massage (1)

Abdominal pain with an aversion to massage (1)

Bad taste in the mouth (2)*

Belching of bad breath after meals (2)*

Chest and diaphragm congestion and discomfort (1)

Diarrhea and constipation (1)

Hiccups with loud and forceful sound (2)*

Hot sensations in the middle of palms (1)

Indigestion (1)

Lack of appetite (1)

Love of hot drink, but drink only a little (1)

Nausea (1)

Pain in inner part of stomach with swelling and feeling of fullness (1)

Stomachache (1)

Stool with an extremely bad smell (1)

Vomiting (1)

Treatment principle: to promote digestion, regulate the stomach, and stop hiccups

Treatment formula: *Bao-He-Wan*

Food cures: asafoetida, buckwheat, castor bean, jellyfish, peach, radish, water chestnut, cardamon seed, cayenne pepper, coriander, grapefruit, jackfruit, malt, sweet basil, tea, and tomato

4. Yin deficiency syndrome ( )

Symptoms:
Bleeding from gums (1)

Constipation (1)

Dizziness (1)

Dry and scant stools (1)

Dry sensations in the mouth (1)

Dry throat (1)

Fatigue (1)

Headache in the afternoon (1)

Hiccups that occur more readily on an empty stomach (2)*

Hiccups with weak and low sound (2)*

Light fever in the afternoon (1)

Night sweats (1)

Nosebleed (1)

Short and reddish streams of urine (1)

Sleeplessness (1)

Swallowing difficulty (1)

Toothache (1)

Underweight (1)

Treatment principle: to produce fluids and strengthen the stomach and to lubricate dryness and stop hiccups

Treatment formula: *Yi-Wei-Tang*
Food cures: bird's nest, cheese,
  kidney bean, abalone, asparagus,
  chicken egg, cuttlefish, duck, duck
  egg, white fungus, oyster, pork,
  and royal jelly

5. Yang deficiency syndrome ( )

Symptoms:
Clear and long streams of urine (1)
Cold hands and feet (1)
Constipation or diarrhea (1)
Diminished urination (1)
Discharge of watery, thin stools (1)
Fatigue (1)
Fear of cold (1)
Fingertips often cold (1)
Frequent fear of cold both in hands
  and feet (1)
Headache in the morning (1)
Hiccups that occur more readily on
  an empty stomach (2)*
Hiccups with weak and low sound
  (3)*
Palpitations (1)
Perspiration due to hot weather or
  putting on warm clothes (1)
Perspiration like cold water (1)
Scant energy and too tired to talk (1)
Sleep a lot (1)
Treatment principle: to tone the
  spleen and the kidneys and to
  harmonize the stomach and stop
  hiccups
Treatment formula: *Li-Zhong Tang*
Food cures: kidneys, lobster, sardine,
  shrimp, star anise, and red and
  black date

CONSTIPATION

1. Large-intestine heat syndrome ( )

Symptoms:
Abdominal pain (2)

Constipation with bad breath (5)*
Discharge of blood from anus (1)
Discharge of solid, dry, and hard
  stools (5)*
Discharge of sticky, muddy stools
  with a rotten and bad smell (1)
Dry sensations in the mouth (1)
Gums swelling (1)
Lips are scorched (1)
Pain in anus with swelling and
  burning sensations (1)
Short and reddish streams of urine
  (1)
Yellow stools like rice pulp with bad
  smell (1)
Treatment principle: to clear heat
  and lubricate the large intestine
Treatment formula: *Ma-Zi-Ren-Wan*
  or *Zeng-Yi-Cheng-Qi-Tang*
Food cures: preserved duck egg,
  flour, banana, bitter endive, black
  fungus, salt, spinach, strawberry,
  bamboo shoot, cucumber, Job's-
  tears, laver, leaf beet, mung bean,
  peppermint, purslane, sesame oil,
  and apple

2. Energy congestion syndrome ( )

Symptoms:
Abdominal pain (2)
Chest and ribs discomfort (1)
Chest pain (2)
Constipation with a desire to empty
  the bowel (5)*
Pain in inner part of stomach with
  prickling sensation and swelling
  (1)
Pain in the upper abdomen (2)
Retention of urine (1)
Ringing in ears and deafness (1)
Stomachache (2)
Subjective sensation of lump in the
  throat (1)
Swallowing difficulty (1)

Swelling and congestion after eating
(1)

Treatment principle: to promote energy flow

Treatment formula: *Liu-Mo-Yin*

Food cures: beef, cherry, bird's nest, butterfish, chicken, coconut meat, date, tofu, mustard seed, sweet rice, goose meat, mutton, jackfruit, squash, sweet potato, red and black date, rice, rock sugar, caraway seed, spearmint, common button mushroom, oregano, red bean, ambergris, dill seed, garlic, sweet basil, and saffron

3. Cold large-intestine syndrome ( )

Symptoms:

Abdominal pain (4)*

Abdominal pain with abdominal rumbling (2)

Abdominal rumbling (2)

Clear and long streams of urine (2)

Cold hands and feet (2)

Difficult bowel movements (5)*

Discharge of sticky, muddy stools not unlike dung of a goose (3)

Treatment principle: to warm the large intestine and promote bowel movements

Treatment formula: *Ji-Chuan-Jian*

Food cures: capers, cayenne pepper, fresh ginger, prickly ash, star anise, white or yellow mustard seed, white or yellow mustard, wine, chicken, clove, herring, nutmeg, and black and white pepper

4. Energy deficiency syndrome ( )

Symptoms:

Abdominal pain (1)

Constipation with discharge of soft stools (1)*

Discharge of sticky, turbid stools or diarrhea (1)*

Dizziness (1)

Fatigued following bowel movement (1)*

Headache (severe) that occurs with fatigue after labor (1)

Headache at intervals, headache in the morning, or prolonged headache (1)

Lying down with an inability to sit up, which will cause dizziness (1)

Misty vision (1)

Numbness (1)

Palpitations with insecure feeling (1)

Perspiration on hands and feet (1)

Prolonged headache (1)

Ringing in ears that causes deafness (1)

Shaking of hands (1)

Shortness of breath (1)

Swallowing difficulty (1)

Talking in weak voice (1)

Tips of four limbs slightly cold (1)

Underweight with dry skin (1)

Treatment principle: to strengthen the energy and promote bowel movement

Treatment formula: *Bu-Zhong-Yi-Qi-Tang*

Food cures: grape, longan nuts, maltose, mandarin fish, Irish potato, sweet rice, apple cucumber, bog bean, gold carp, carrot, chestnut, ham, horse bean, hyacinth bean, Job's-tears, royal jelly, string bean, whitefish, yam, red and black date, mutton, squash, and rock sugar

5. Blood deficiency syndrome ( )

Symptoms:

Abdominal pain (1)

Constipation with discharge of hard stool (1)*
Difficult bowel movement (1)*
Dizziness (1)
Dry and cracked lips and mouth (1)
Fatigue (1)
Fever (1)
Feeling miserable (1)
Headache in the afternoon or with dizziness (1)
Lips lightly colored (1)
Lying down with an inability to sit up, which will cause dizziness (1)
Misty vision (1)
Muscles jumping that cannot be controlled (1)
Night sweats (1)
Palpitations with insecure feeling (1)
Sleeplessness (1)
Spasms (1)
Tics of four limbs (1)
Underweight with dry skin (1)
White complexion (1)
Treatment principle: to nourish the blood and lubricate the large intestine
Treatment formula: *Run-Chang-Wan*
Food cures: abalone, asparagus, cuttlefish, chicken egg, duck egg, white fungus, beef liver, grape, mandarin fish, oyster, milk, beef, cherry, blood clam, and longan nuts

DIARRHEA

1. Cold-dampness syndrome ( )

Symptoms:
Absence of perspiration in hot weather (1)
Cold sensations in lower abdomen–genitals region (1)
Cough (1)
Coughing out sputum with a low sound (1)

Diarrhea with discharge of soft stools with an offensive smell (6)*
Discharge of sputum that can be coughed out easily (1)
Dysentery (2)
Edema in the four limbs (1)
Headache (1)
Movement difficulty (1)
Pain in the body (1)
Pain in the joints (1)
Scant and clear urine (1)
Stomachache (1)
Treatment principle: to remove dampness with aromatic herbs and to disperse cold and dry dampness
Treatment formula: *Huo-Xiang-Zheng-Qi-San*
Food cures: cayenne pepper, dill seed, fennel, fresh ginger, mustard seed, prickly ash, star anise, white or yellow mustard, wine, carp, celery, horse bean, jellyfish skin, Job's-tears, hyacinth bean, oregano, sweet basil, adzuki bean, bamboo shoot, soybean sprouts, and rosin

2. Superficial dampness-heat syndrome ( )

Symptoms:
Burning sensation and itch in the genitals or burning sensation in the anus (1)
Diarrhea with forceful discharge of stools (5)*
Discharge of yellowish-red, turbid stools with bad smell (1)
Excessive perspiration (1)
Feeling miserable (1)
Itch and pain in the vulva frequently (1)
Low fever (1)
Pain in the joints of four limbs, with swelling and heaviness (1)

Paralysis (1)
Perspiration on hands and feet or the head (1)
Reddish and scant streams of urine (1)
Retention of urine (1)
Short and reddish streams of urine (1)
Swollen body of the tongue (1)
Thirst (1)
Yellowish color of body (1)
Treatment principle: to clear heat and remove dampness and to regulate the stomach and the intestine
Treatment formula: *Ge-Gen-Qin-Lian-Tang*
Food cures: carp, celery, horse bean, jellyfish skin, Job's-tears, prickly ash, hyacinth bean, oregano, sweet basil, adzuki bean, bamboo shoot, soybean sprouts, rosin, banana, bitter endive, black fungus, salt, spinach, strawberry, cucumber, leaf beet, mung bean, peppermint, and purslane

3. Indigestion syndrome (   )

Symptoms:
Abdominal pain that lessens following bowel movement (3)*
Belching of bad breath after meals (1)
Chest and diaphragm congestion and discomfort (1)
Diarrhea and constipation (1)
Diarrhea with an unusually offensive smell (3)*
Hot sensations in the middle of palms (1)
Indigestion (1)
Lack of appetite (1)
Love of hot drink, but drink only a little (1)
Malaria (1)

Nausea (1)
Pain in inner part of stomach with swelling and feeling of fullness (1)
Stomachache (1)
Stools with an extremely bad smell (1)
Vomiting (1)
Vomiting of clear water (1)
Treatment principle: to promote digestion and regulate the stomach and intestine
Treatment formula: *Mu-Xiang-Bing-Lang-Wan*
Food cures: asafoetida, buckwheat, castor bean, jellyfish, peach, radish, water chestnut, cardamon seed, cayenne pepper, coriander, grapefruit, jackfruit, malt, sweet basil, tea, and tomato

4. Liver offending the spleen Syndrome (   )

Symptoms:
Abdominal enlargement (3)
Abdominal pain (3)
Abdominal rumbling (1)
Chronic diarrhea (1)
Diarrhea occurs right after abdominal pain starts (8)*
Fatigued spirits (1)
Hungry with no appetite (2)
Thirst with no desire for drink (1)
Treatment principle: to regulate energy and oppress the liver and to harmonize the stomach and support the spleen
Treatment formula: *Tong-Xie-Yao-Fang*
Food cures: brown sugar, kumquat, mandarin orange, apple cucumber, bog bean, gold carp, carrot, chestnut, corncob, horse bean, hyacinth bean, Job's-tears, Irish potato, royal jelly, string bean, whitefish, and yam

5. Spleen-dampness syndrome ( )

Symptoms:
Chest discomfort without appetite (1)
Diarrhea that comes and goes (5)*
Diarrhea with discharge of watery stools (5)*
Edema (1)
Heavy sensations in head as if the head were covered with something (1)
Heavy sensations in the body with discomfort (1)
Jaundice (1)
Love of hot drink (1)
Nausea and vomiting (1)
Stomach fullness and discomfort (1)
Sweet, sticky taste in mouth (1)
Too tired to talk or move (1)
Treatment principle: to tone the energy and strengthen the spleen and to help dampness seep and stop diarrhea
Treatment formula: *Shen-Ling-Bai-Zhu-San* or *Bu-Zhong-Yi-Qi-Tang*
Food cures: gold carp, corncob, horse bean, Job's-tears, prickly ash, adzuki bean, and bamboo shoot

6. Spleen-kidneys yang deficiency syndrome ( )

Symptoms:
Ascites (1)
Being physically weak and too tired to talk (1)
Cold hands and feet (1)
Cold loins (1)
Diarrhea before dawn (2)*
Diarrhea right after pain occurs (2)*
Diarrhea with sticky and muddy stools (1)
Dysentery (1)
Eating only a little (1)

Edema (1)
Edema that occurs all over the body (1)
Fatigue (1)
Fear of cold (1)
Feeling comfortable after bowel movement (1)
Four limbs weakness (1)
Frequent urination with clear or white urine (1)
Mentally fatigued (1)
Sputum rumbling with panting (1)
Treatment principle: to warm the spleen and the kidneys and to solidify the intestine and stop diarrhea
Treatment formula: *Si-Shen-Wan*
Food cures: air bladder of shark, chicken, cayenne pepper, fennel, nutmeg, black and white pepper, prickly ash, mutton, sword bean, white or yellow mustard, kidney, lobster, sardine, shrimp, sparrow, clove, dill seed, fennel, pistachio nut, sparrow egg, crab apple, raspberry, and walnut

CHEST PAIN

1. Cold syndrome ( )

Symptoms:
Abdominal pain (1)
Absence of perspiration in hot weather (1)
Absence of thirst in mouth (1)
Abundant watering of eyes (1)
Chest pain that affects the back of shoulders (1)
Chest pain often triggered or intensified by cold (2)*
Clear and long streams of urine in large amounts (1)
Cold chest, cold hands and feet, or cold bodily sensations (1)
Constipation (1)

Contraction of tendons and muscles (1)
Diarrhea with watery stools containing undigested food or with sticky and muddy stools (1)
Dizziness with objects appearing in front of eyes (1)
Dry throat (1)
Hands and feet extremely cold (1)
Heavy and unclear voice in high-pitched and rough tone (1)
Hiccups with cold hands and feet and mild taste in mouth, triggered by cold air (1)
Love of hot drink (1)
Pain in the throat (1)
Pain shifting around with no fixed region (1)
Pale complexion (1)
Perspire heavily (1)
Treatment principle: to warm the internal region and disperse cold
Treatment formula: *Zhi-Gan-Cao-Tang* or *Gua-Lou-Xie-Bai-Bai-Jiu-Tang*
Food cures: cayenne pepper, dill seed, fennel, fresh ginger, mustard seed, prickly ash, star anise, white or yellow mustard, and wine

2. Dampness-sputum syndrome ( )

Symptoms:
Chest pain that affects the back of shoulders (3)*
Chest pain that is dull and mild (2)*
Cough (2)
Discharge of sputum that can be coughed out easily (1)
Discharge of white, watery sputum (1)
Dizziness (1)
Headache (1)
Hiccups (1)
Panting (2)

Prolonged dizziness (1)
Sleep a lot (1)
Sleeplessness (1)
Vomiting (2)
White, sliding sputum that can be cleared from throat easily (1)
Treatment principle: to transform sputum and remove dampness
Treatment formula: *Gua-Lou-Xie-Bai-Ban-Xia-Tang*
Food cures: adzuki bean, ambergris, barley, common carp, cucumber, mung bean, seaweed, shepherd's purse, star fruit, bamboo shoot, crown daisy, date, fresh ginger, leaf or brown mustard, black and white pepper, white or yellow mustard seed, asparagus, and pear

3. Blood coagulations syndrome ( )

Symptoms:
Abdominal pain (1)
Chest pain in a fixed region without shifting around (2)*
Chest pain that is caused by injuries (2)*
Chest pain that worsens on pressure (2)*
Coughing up blood (1)
Pain in the upper abdomen (1)
Palpitations with insecure feeling (2)*
Partial suppression of lochia (1)
Spasm (2)*
Stomachache (2)*
Stroke (2)*
Swelling and congestion after eating (1)
Vomiting of blood (1)
Treatment principle: to remove blood coagulations and promote blood circulation
Treatment formula: *Shen-Tong-Zhu-Yu-Tang*
Food cures: ambergris, brown sugar, chestnut, eggplant, peach, black

soybean, sturgeon, sweet basil, crab, distillers' grains, papaya, and saffron

PAIN IN THE UPPER ABDOMEN

1. Wind-cold syndrome (   )

Symptoms:
Absence of perspiration in hot weather (1)
Clear discharge from nose (1)
Cough (1)
Diarrhea (1)
Dislike of cold (1)
Dizziness (1)
Facial paralysis (1)
Fever or hot and cold sensations that come and go (1)
Headache (1)
Headache with dizziness (1)
Hoarseness at the beginning of illness (1)
Loss of voice (1)
Nausea (1)
Nosebleed (1)
Pain in the body shifting around with no fixed region (1)
Pain in the upper abdomen with chest congestion (2)*
Pain in the joints (1)
Stuffed nose (1)
Vomiting (1)
Treatment principle: to reduce the heat in the gallbladder
Treatment formula: *Xiao-Chai-Hu-Tang*
Food cures: peppermint (including oil), spearmint, sweet basil, cayenne pepper, fennel, fresh ginger, mustard seed, star anise, and prickly ash leaf

2. Superficial dampness-heat syndrome (   )

Symptoms:
Abdominal pain (1)

Burning sensation and itch in the genitals or burning sensation in the anus (1)
Congested chest (1)
Diarrhea with forceful discharge of stools (1)
Discharge of yellowish-red, turbid stools with bad smell (1)
Edema (1)
Excessive perspiration (1)
Itch and pain in the vulva frequently (1)
Jaundice (1)
Low fever (1)
Pain in the upper abdomen that worsens with massage (2)*
Pain in the joints of the four limbs, with swelling and heaviness (1)
Perspiration on hands and feet or the head (1)
Reddish and scant urine (1)
Retention of urine (1)
Severe pain in the upper abdomen (2)*
Short streams of reddish urine (1)
Swollen body of the tongue (1)
Thirst (1)
Treatment principle: to clear dampness-heat in the liver and the gallbladder
Treatment formula: *Yin-Chen-Hao-Tang* or *Long-Dan-Xie-Gan-Tang*
Food cures: carp, celery, horse bean, jellyfish skin, Job's-tears, prickly ash, hyacinth bean, oregano, sweet basil, adzuki bean, bamboo shoot, soybean sprouts, rosin, banana, bitter endive, black fungus, salt, spinach, strawberry, cucumber, leaf beet, mung bean, peppermint, and purslane

3. Liver-fire upsurging syndrome (   )

Symptoms:
Acute dizziness (1)

Bleeding from stomach (1)
Deafness (1)
Dim vision (1)
Dizziness (1)
Dry sensations in the mouth (1)
Getting angry easily (1)
Headache on both sides of the head
    and in the corners of the eyes (1)
Headache that is severe (1)
Hiccups (1)
Nosebleed (1)
Pain (falling) in the lower abdomen
    with desire for massage (1)
Pain in the chest and the ribs (1)
Pain in the upper abdomen triggered
    by anger or emotional upset (1)*
Pink eyes with swelling (1)
Red eyes (1)
Ringing in ears (1)
Severe pain in the upper abdomen
    (1)*
Sleeplessness or sleep a lot (1)
Vomiting of blood (1)
Treatment principle: to calm the
    liver and sedate fire in the liver
Treatment formula: *Qing-Gan-Tang*
Food cures: spinach, chestnut,
    shepherd's purse, rye, black
    fungus, vinegar, abalone,
    asparagus, chicken egg, white
    fungus, pork, and royal jelly

4. Energy congestion syndrome ( )

Symptoms:
Abdominal pain (2)
Chest and ribs discomfort (1)
Chest pain (2)
Constipation with a desire to empty
    the bowel (3)*
Pain in inner part of stomach with
    pricking sensations and swelling
    (1)
Pain in the upper abdomen that
    moves around (3)*

Poor appetite (1)
Retention of urine (1)
Ringing in ears and deafness (1)
Stomachache (2)
Subjective sensation of lump in the
    throat (1)
Swallowing difficulty (1)
Swelling and congestion after eating
    (1)
Treatment principle: to relax the
    liver and regulate the energy of
    the liver and to strengthen the
    spleen and nourish the blood
Treatment formula: *Xiao-Yao-San* or
    Chai-Hu-Shu-Gan-San
Food cures: beef, cherry, bird's nest,
    butterfish, chicken, coconut meat,
    date, tofu, mustard seed, sweet
    rice, goose meat, mutton, jackfruit,
    squash, sweet potato, red and
    black date, rice, rock sugar,
    caraway seed, spearmint, common
    button mushroom, oregano, red
    bean, ambergris, dill seed, garlic,
    sweet basil, saffron, sweet potato,
    red and black date, Chinese chive,
    brown sugar, mandarin orange,
    and garlic

5. Blood coagulations syndrome ( )

Symptoms:
Abdominal pain (1)
Bleeding from gums (1)
Chest pain (1)
Coughing out blood (1)
Headache (1)
Jaundice (1)
Lumbago (1)
Pain in the upper abdomen as if
    being pricked by a sharp needle
    (2)*
Pain in the upper abdomen in a fixed
    region without moving around (2)*
Pain in the loins as if being pierced
    with an awl (1)

Pain in the ribs (1)
Palpitations with insecure feeling (1)
Partial suppression of lochia (1)
Spasm (1)
Stomachache (1)
Stroke (1)
Swelling and congestion after eating (1)
Vomiting of blood (1)
Treatment principle: to transform blood coagulations and regulate energy
Treatment formula: *Ge-Xia-Zhu-Yu-Tang*
Food cures: ambergris, brown sugar, chestnut, eggplant, peach, black soybean, sturgeon, sweet basil, crab, distillers' grains, papaya, and saffron

6. Dampness syndrome ( )

Symptoms:
Abdominal pain with abdominal rumbling (1)
Diarrhea (1)
Diminished urination (1)
Discharge of hard stool followed by sticky, turbid stool (1)
Dizziness (1)
Headache as if the head were being wrapped up (1)
Heavy sensation in body with intestinal rumbling and watery stools (1)
Heavy sensations and stagnation of lower limbs (1)
Heavy sensations in head as if head were wrapped up (1)
Heavy sensations in the body (1)
Illness starts mostly from lower regions of the body (1)
Itch (1)
Love of hot drink (1)
Love of sleep and heavy sensations in the body (1)

Pain always in same joints with heavy sensations in the body (1)
Pain in the loins as if sitting in water with heaviness in body (1)
Quick bowel movements (1)
Stomach and abdomen swollen and full (1)
Toes extremely itchy (1)
White, small granular pimples in the skin (1)
Treatment principle: to strengthen the spleen, dry dampness, and regulate the liver
Treatment formula: *Bu-Huan-Jin-Zheng-Qi-San* or *Shen-Ling-Bai-Zhu-San*
Food cures: carp, celery, horse bean, jellyfish skin, Job's-tears, prickly ash, hyacinth bean, oregano, sweet basil, adzuki bean, bamboo shoot, soybean sprouts, and rosin

7. Yin deficiency syndrome ( )

Symptoms:
Bleeding from gums (1)
Constipation (1)
Dizziness (1)
Dry and scant stool (1)
Dry sensations in the mouth (1)
Dry throat (1)
Fatigue (2)
Headache in the afternoon (1)
Jaundice (1)
Light fever in the afternoon (1)
Night sweats (1)
Nosebleed (1)
Pain in the throat, also red and swollen (1)
Palms of hands and soles of feet are both hot (1)
Palpitations with insecure feeling (1)
Severe pain in the body that attacks all of a sudden (1)
Short streams of reddish urine (1)

Sleeplessness (1)
Swallowing difficulty (1)
Toothache (1)
Underweight (1)
Treatment principle: to water the yin and nourish the blood and to soften up the liver
Treatment formula: *Yi-Guan-Jian* or *Liu-Wei-Di-Huang-Wan*
Food cures: bird's nest, cheese, kidney bean, abalone, asparagus, chicken egg, cuttlefish, duck, duck egg, white fungus, oyster, pork, and royal jelly

STOMACHACHE

1. Liver energy congestion syndrome ( )

Symptoms:
Abdominal obstruction (2)
Abdominal pain (2)
Belching (1)
Convulsions (1)
Nausea (1)
Numbness (1)
Stomachache that affects the upper abdomen and gets slightly better with massage (5)*
Stomachache that worsens with anger (6)*
Subjective sensations of objects in the throat (3)
Vomiting of blood (1)
Treatment principle: to disperse energy congestion, regulate energy conditions, and harmonize the stomach and relieve pain
Treatment formula: *Si-Ni-San*
Food cures: brown sugar, garlic, turmeric, kumquat, beef, cherry, bird's nest, butterfish, chicken, coconut meat, date, tofu, mustard seed, sweet rice, goose meat, mutton, jackfruit, squash, sweet potato, red and black date, rice, rock sugar, caraway seed, spearmint, common button mushroom, oregano, red bean, ambergris, dill seed, garlic, sweet basil, and saffron

2. Blood coagulations syndrome ( )

Symptoms:
Abdominal pain (1)
Bleeding from gums (1)
Chest pain (1)
Coughing out blood (1)
Headache (1)
Jaundice (1)
Lumbago (1)
Pain (acute) around umbilicus resisting massage, and hard spots felt by hands (1)
Pain in region between navel and pubic hair with feeling of hardness (1)
Pain in the upper abdomen as if being pricked by a needle (1)
Pain in the upper abdomen that worsens after eating (2)*
Pain in the loins as if being pierced with an awl (1)
Pain in the ribs (1)
Palpitations with insecure feeling (1)
Spasm (1)
Stomachache (1)
Stroke (1)
Swelling and congestion after eating (1)
Vomiting of blood (1)
Treatment principle: to activate the blood and transform coagulations and to harmonize the stomach and relieve pain
Treatment formula: *Shi-Xiao-San*
Food cures: ambergris, brown sugar, chestnut, eggplant, peach, black soybean, sturgeon, sweet basil,

crab, distillers' grains, papaya, and saffron

3. Indigestion syndrome (   )

Symptoms:
Abdominal pain (1)
Belching of bad breath after meals (1)
Chest and diaphragm congestion and discomfort (1)
Diarrhea and constipation (1)
Diarrhea in children (1)
Hot sensations in the middle of palms (1)
Indigestion (1)
Lack of appetite (1)
Love of hot drink, but drink only a little (1)
Malaria (1)
Nausea (1)
Pain in inner part of stomach with swelling and feeling of fullness (1)
Stomachache that worsens with massage (2)*
Stomachache that occurs all of a sudden with dislike of foods (3)*
Stools with an extremely bad smell(1)
Vomiting (1)
Vomiting of clear water (1)
Treatment principle: to promote digestion and harmonize the stomach
Treatment formula: *Bao-He-Wan*
Food cures: asafoetida, buckwheat, castor bean, jellyfish, peach, radish, water chestnut, cardamon seed, cayenne pepper, coriander, grapefruit, jackfruit, malt, sweet basil, tea, and tomato

4. Deficiency and cold syndrome (   )

Symptoms:
Abdominal pain on the right and left sides of navel (umbilicus)
Cold hands and feet (2)
Cold sensations in lower abdomen–genitals region (1)
Diarrhea containing undigested food (2)
Fatigue (1)
Fear of cold (2)
Fingerprint appears light red (1)
Love of hot drink (3)*
Love of sighing (1)
Night sweats (1)
Palpitations (1)
Run-down feeling (1)
Shortness of breath (1)
Vomiting slowly with a feeble sound (1)
White complexion (1)
Treatment principle: to strengthen the spleen and the stomach and to warm the internal region and disperse cold
Treatment formula: *Li-Zhong-Tang* or *Xiang-Sha-Liu-Jun-Zi-Tang*
Food cures: cayenne pepper, dill seed, fennel, fresh ginger, mustard seed, prickly ash, star anise, white or yellow mustard, wine, grape, longan nuts, maltose, mandarin fish, Irish potato, sweet rice, apple cucumber, bog bean, gold carp, carrot, chestnut, ham, horse bean, hyacinth bean, Job's-tears, royal jelly, string bean, whitefish, yam, red and black date, mutton, squash, and rock sugar

5. Yin deficiency syndrome (   )

Symptoms:
Bleeding from gums (1)
Burning pain in the stomach (1)
Constipation (1)
Dry and scant stools (1)
Dry sensations in the mouth (1)
Dry throat (1)

Fatigue (1)
Headache in the afternoon (1)
Light fever in the afternoon (1)
Night sweats (1)
Nosebleed (1)
Pain in the throat (1)
Pain in the throat, also red and
    swollen (1)
Palms of hands and soles of feet are
    both hot (1)
Short streams of reddish urine (1)
Sleeplessness (1)
Stomachache that worsens when the
    stomach is empty (2)*
Toothache (1)
Underweight (1)
Treatment principle: to tone the yin
    and strengthen the stomach and
    to clear the heat in the stomach
Treatment formula: *Mai-Men-Dong-
    Tang*
Food cures: bird's nest, cheese,
    kidney bean, abalone, asparagus,
    chicken egg, cuttlefish, duck, duck
    egg, white fungus, oyster, pork,
    and royal jelly

ABDOMINAL PAIN

1. Cold spleen syndrome (　)

Symptoms:
Abdominal pain that attacks all of a
    sudden (3)*
Abdominal pain that drags on and on
    (1)
Abdominal pain that gets worse
    when cold and better when warm
    (4)*
Cold hands and feet (1)
Dark-yellow skin (1)
Diarrhea with a feeling of coolness
    (1)
Discharge of watery, thin stools (1)
Edema (1)

Indigestion (1)
Lips lightly colored (1)
Pleasant taste in the mouth (1)
Poor appetite (1)
Prolonged diarrhea (1)
Runny, thin saliva (1)
Vomiting (1)
Treatment principle: to disperse cold
    and warm the spleen
Treatment formula: *Wen-Pi-Tang*
Food cures: cinnamon, clove oil, dill
    seed, garlic, pistachio nut, cayenne
    pepper, fennel, fresh ginger,
    mustard seed, prickly ash, star
    anise, white or yellow mustard,
    and wine

2. Deficiency and cold syndrome (　)

Symptoms:
Abdominal pain that drags on and on
    (2)*
Abdominal pain that gets worse
    when cold and better when warm
    (2)*
Abdominal pain that gets worse
    when hungry (3)*
Cold hands and feet (1)
Cold sensations in lower abdomen–
    genitals region (1)
Diarrhea containing undigested food
    (1)
Fatigue (1)
Fear of cold (1)
Love of hot drink (1)
Love of sighing (1)
Night sweats (1)
Palpitations (1)
Run-down feeling (1)
Shortness of breath (1)
Vomiting slowly with a feeble sound
    (1)
White complexion (1)

Treatment principle: to strengthen energy and warm the internal region

Treatment formula: *Li-Zhong-Tang*

Food cures: cayenne pepper, dill seed, fennel, fresh ginger, mustard seed, prickly ash, star anise, white or yellow mustard, wine, grape, longan nuts, maltose, mandarin fish, Irish potato, sweet rice, apple cucumber, bog bean, gold carp, carrot, chestnut, ham, horse bean, hyacinth bean, Job's-tears, royal jelly, string bean, whitefish, yam, red and black date, mutton, squash, and rock sugar

3. Excess and hot syndrome ( )

Symptoms:

Abdominal pain that gets worse when hot and better when cold (6)*

Abdominal pain that gets worse with massage (5)*

Abdominal pain with burning sensations (5)*

Constant desire for drink, but drink only a little (1)

Hiccups that make loud and forceful sound (1)

Pain in the throat, also red and swollen (1)

Vomiting that comes on rather forcefully, with a strong sound (1)

Treatment principle: to sedate heat and regulate energy

Treatment formula: *Hou-Pu-San-Wu-Tang*

Food cures: banana, bitter endive, black fungus, salt, spinach, strawberry, bamboo shoot, cucumber, Job's-tears, laver, leaf beet, mung bean, peppermint, and purslane

4. Indigestion syndrome ( )

Symptoms:

Abdominal pain that gets worse with massage and better after bowel movement (4)*

Belching of bad breath after meals (1)

Diarrhea and constipation (1)

Dislike of foods (1)

Hot sensations in the middle of palms (1)

Indigestion (1)

Lack of appetite (1)

Love of hot drink, but drink only a little (1)

Nausea (1)

Pain in inner part of stomach with swelling and feeling of fullness (1)

Stomachache (4)*

Stools with an extremely bad smell (1)

Vomiting (1)

Vomiting of clear water (1)

Treatment principle: to promote digestion and harmonize the stomach

Treatment formula: *Bao-He-Wan* or *Zhi-Shi-Dao-Zhi-Wan*

Food cures: asafoetida, buckwheat, castor bean, jellyfish, peach, radish, water chestnut, cardamon seed, cayenne pepper, coriander, grapefruit, jackfruit, malt, sweet basil, tea, and tomato

5. Energy congestion syndrome ( )

Symptoms:

Abdominal pain that reduces after flatulence (2)*

Belching or hiccups (2)*

Chest and ribs discomfort (1)

Chest pain (1)

Constipation with a desire to empty the bowel (2)*
Pain in inner part of stomach with prickling sensation and swelling (1)
Pain in the upper abdomen (2)*
Retention of urine (1)
Ringing in ears and deafness (1)
Stomachache (2)*
Subjective sensation of lump in the throat (1)
Swallowing difficulty (1)
Swelling and congestion after eating (1)
Treatment principle: to regulate energy and promote energy circulation
Treatment formula: *Mu-Xiang-Shun-Qi-San*
Food cures: beef, cherry, bird's nest, butterfish, chicken, coconut meat, date, tofu, mustard seed, sweet rice, goose meat, mutton, jackfruit, squash, sweet potato, red and black date, rice, rock sugar, caraway seed, spearmint, common button mushroom, oregano, red bean, ambergris, dill seed, garlic, sweet basil, and saffron

6. Blood coagulations syndrome ( )

Symptoms:
Abdominal pain as if being pricked by a needle (2)*
Abdominal pain in a fixed region without moving around (1)
Bleeding from gums (1)
Chest pain (1)
Coughing out blood (1)
Headache (1)
Jaundice (1)
Lumbago (1)
Pain (acute) around umbilicus resisting massage, and hard spots felt by hands (1)

Pain in region between navel and pubic hair with feeling of hardness (1)
Pain in the upper abdomen (1)
Pain in the loins as if being pierced with an awl (1)
Pain in the ribs (1)
Palpitations with insecure feeling (1)
Spasm (1)
Stomachache (1)
Stroke (1)
Swelling and congestion after eating (1)
Vomiting of blood (1)
Treatment principle: to activate the blood and transform coagulations and to promote energy circulation and relieve pain
Treatment formula: *Shao-Fu-Zhu-Yu-Tang*
Food cures: ambergris, brown sugar, chestnut, eggplant, peach, black soybean, sturgeon, sweet basil, crab, distillers' grains, papaya, and saffron

LUMBAGO (LOWER-BACK PAIN)

1. Wind-dampness syndrome ( )

Symptoms:
Chronic backache (1)
Diarrhea (1)
Eczema (1)
Edema (1)
Fever that becomes more severe in the afternoon (1)
German measles (1)
Headache with heavy sensations in the head (1)
Itchy sores (1)
Light swelling (1)
Lower-back pain affecting the lower limbs (4)*

Lower-back pain that gets worse on rainy days (4)*

Pain in all the joints (1)

Pain shifting around with no fixed region (1)

Scant urine (1)

Treatment principle: to expel wind and disperse cold and to remove dampness and relieve pain

Treatment formula: *Du-Huo-Ji-Sheng-Tang*

Food cures: peppermint, spearmint, sweet basil, celery, coconut meat, green onion, jellyfish skin, prickly ash, rice, adzuki bean, rosin, and tangerine

2. Cold-dampness syndrome ( )

Symptoms:

Absence of perspiration in hot weather (1)

Cold lower-back pain (5)*

Cold sensations in lower abdomen–genitals region (1)

Cough (1)

Coughing out sputum with a low sound (1)

Diarrhea (2)

Discharge of sputum that can be coughed out easily (1)

Dysentery (2)

Edema in the four limbs (1)

Headache (1)

Movement difficulty particularly in turning around (1)

Pain in the body or in the joints (1)

Scant and clear urine (1)

Stomachache (1)

Treatment principle: to expel cold and remove dampness and to warm the internal region

Treatment formula: *Shen-Zhuo-Tang*

Food cures: cayenne pepper, dill seed, fennel, fresh ginger, mustard seed, prickly ash, star anise, white or yellow mustard, wine, carp, celery, horse bean, jellyfish skin, Job's-tears, hyacinth bean, oregano, sweet basil, adzuki bean, bamboo shoot, soybean sprouts, and rosin

3. Superficial dampness-heat syndrome ( )

Symptoms:

Abdominal pain (1)

Burning sensation and itch in the genitals or burning sensation in the anus (1)

Congested chest (1)

Diarrhea with forceful discharge of stools (1)*

Discharge of yellowish-red, turbid stools with bad smell (1)

Edema (1)

Excessive perspiration (1)

Feeling miserable (1)

Jaundice (1)

Low fever (1)

Lower-back pain with a weak back or burning sensations (1)*

Pain in the joints of four limbs, with swelling and heaviness (1)

Paralysis (1)

Perspiration on hands and feet or the head (1)

Reddish and scant urine (1)

Retention of urine (1)

Short streams of reddish urine (1)

Swollen body of the tongue (1)

Thirst (1)

Yellowish color of body (1)

Treatment principle: to clear heat and remove dampness and to promote energy circulation

Treatment formula: *San-Miao-Wan*

Food cures: carp, celery, horse bean, jellyfish skin, Job's-tears, prickly ash, hyacinth bean, oregano, sweet basil, adzuki bean, bamboo shoot, soybean sprouts, rosin, banana, bitter endive, black fungus, salt, spinach, strawberry, cucumber, leaf beet, mung bean, peppermint, and purslane

4. Blood coagulations syndrome (   )

Symptoms:
Abdominal pain (1)
Bleeding from gums (1)
Chest pain (1)
Coughing out blood (1)
Headache (1)
Jaundice (1)
Lower-back pain as sharp as being cut by a knife (1)*
Lower-back pain that worsens with massage (1)*
Lower-back pain that occurs in a fixed region without moving around (1)*
Pain (acute) around umbilicus resisting massage, and hard spots felt by hands (1)
Pain in region between navel and pubic hair with feeling of hardness (1)
Pain in the upper abdomen (1)
Pain in the loins as if being pierced with an awl (1)
Pain in the ribs (1)
Palpitations with insecure feeling (1)
Partial suppression of lochia (1)
Spasm (1)
Stomachache (1)
Stroke (1)
Swelling and congestion after eating (1)
Vomiting of blood (1)
Treatment principle: to activate the blood and transform coagulations and to regulate energy and relieve pain

Treatment formula: *Shen-Tong-Zhu-Yu-Tang*
Food cures: ambergris, brown sugar, chestnut, eggplant, peach, black soybean, sturgeon, sweet basil, crab, distillers' grains, papaya, and saffron

5. Kidneys yin deficiency syndrome (   )

Symptoms:
Cold hands and feet (1)
Cough with sputum containing blood or coughing out fresh blood (1)
Dizziness (1)
Dry sensations in the mouth (1)
Dry throat (1)
Fatigue (1)
Feeling miserable and hurried, with fever (1)
Hot sensations in body (1)
Hot sensations in the middle of palms or soles of feet (1)
Lower-back pain that drags on and on (1)*
Lower-back pain that worsens with fatigue (1)*
Lower-back pain with weakness of the back (1)*
Night sweats (1)
Pain in the heels (1)
Retention of urine (1)
Ringing in ears (1)
Seminal emission with dreams (1)
Sleeplessness (1)
Spots in front of the eyes (1)
Thirst (1)
Treatment principle: to tone the yin and clear fire and to nourish the blood
Treatment formula: *Zuo-Gui-Yin*
Food cures: abalone, asparagus, chicken egg, cuttlefish, duck, duck egg, white fungus, oyster, pork, royal jelly, chestnut, chicken liver, and pork kidneys

6. Kidneys yang deficiency syndrome (   )

Symptoms:
Cold feet, cold loins and legs, cold sensations in the genitals, or cold sensations in the muscles (1)
Cough and panting (1)
Diarrhea before dawn (1)
Diarrhea with sticky, muddy stools (1)
Discharge of watery, thin stools (1)
Dizziness (1)
Edema (1)
Fatigue (1)
Frequent urination at night (1)
Impotence (1)
Infertility (1)
Lack of appetite (1)
Panting (1)
Perspiration on the forehead (1)
Retention of urine (1)
Ringing in ears (1)
Seminal emission (1)
Shaky teeth (1)
Shortness of breath (1)
Swelling of body (1)
Wheezing (1)
Treatment principle: to warm the kidney yang
Treatment formula: *You-Gui-Yin*
Food cures: kidney, lobster, sardine, shrimp, sparrow, clove, dill seed, fennel, pistachio nut, sparrow egg, crab apple, raspberry, and walnut

JAUNDICE

1. Superficial dampness-heat syndrome with more heat than dampness (   )

Symptoms:
Abdominal pain (1)
Burning sensation and itch in the genitals or burning sensation in the anus (1)
Congested chest (1)
Diarrhea with forceful discharge of stools (1)
Discharge of dry stools (2)*
Edema (1)
Excessive perspiration (1)
Feeling miserable (1)
Hot sensations in the body (2)*
Low fever (1)
Pain in the joints of four limbs, with swelling and heaviness (1)
Perspiration on hands and feet or the head (1)
Reddish and scant urine (2)*
Retention of urine (1)
Short streams of reddish urine (1)
Thirst (2)*
Treatment principle: to clear heat, sedate fire, remove dampness, and relax the liver
Treatment formula: *Yin-Chen-Hao-Tang*
Food cures: carp, celery, horse bean, jellyfish skin, Job's-tears, prickly ash, hyacinth bean, oregano, sweet basil, adzuki bean, bamboo shoot, soybean sprouts, rosin, banana, bitter endive, black fungus, salt, spinach, strawberry, cucumber, leaf beet, mung bean, peppermint, and purslane

2. Superficial dampness-heat syndrome with more dampness than heat (   )

Symptoms:
Abdominal pain (1)
Burning sensation and itch in the genitals or burning sensation in the anus (2)*
Diarrhea with forceful discharge of stools (2)*
Discharge of watery stools (2)*
Edema (1)
Excessive perspiration (1)

89

Heavy sensations in the body (2)*
Itch and pain in the vulva frequently (1)
Low fever (1)
No thirst (2)*
Pain in the joints of the four limbs, with swelling and heaviness (1)
Perspiration on hands and feet or the head (1)
Poor appetite (2)*
Retention of urine (1)
Treatment principle: to remove dampness and clear heat
Treatment formula: *Yin-Chen-Wu-Ling-San*
Food cures: carp, celery, horse bean, jellyfish skin, Job's-tears, prickly ash, hyacinth bean, oregano, sweet basil, adzuki bean, bamboo shoot, soybean sprouts, rosin, banana, bitter endive, black fungus, salt, spinach, strawberry, cucumber, leaf beet, mung bean, peppermint, and purslane

3. Hot syndrome ( )

Symptoms:
Acute jaundice (2)*
Both the body and eyes are fresh yellowish color (2)*
Burning sensation and itch in the genitals (1)
Constipation (1)
Discharge of blood from the anus (2)*
Dry lips or dry teeth (1)
High fever (2)*
Limbs are warm (1)
Love of cold drink (1)
Nosebleed (2)*
Pain in inner part of stomach becoming acute after meals, and fond of cold (1)
Psychological depression (1)
Reddish complexion, eyes, or urine (1)

Stools with an extremely bad smell (1)
Thirst with an incessant desire to drink (1)
Urine with an extremely bad smell (1)
Treatment principle: to clear toxic heat, cool the blood, and rescue the yin
Treatment formula: *Qian-Jin-Xi-Jiao-San* or *Ju-Fang-Zhi-Bao-Dan*
Food cures: banana, bitter endive, black fungus, salt, spinach, strawberry, bamboo shoot, cucumber, Job's-tears, laver, leaf beet, mung bean, peppermint, and purslane

4. Cold-dampness syndrome ( )

Symptoms:
Absence of perspiration in hot weather (1)
Body and eyes in dark-yellowish color (5)*
Clear urine (1)
Cough (1)
Coughing out sputum with a low sound (1)
Diarrhea (2)
Discharge of sputum that can be coughed out easily (1)
Dysentery (1)
Edema in the four limbs (1)
Headache (1)
Movement difficulty (1)
Pain in the body (1)
Pain in the joints (1)
Soft stools (1)
Stomachache (1)
Treatment principle: to warm the yang and expel dampness and to relax the liver and transform blood coagulations
Treatment formula: *Yin-Chen-Zhu-Fu-Tang*

Food cures: cayenne pepper, dill seed, fennel, fresh ginger, mustard seed, prickly ash, star anise, white or yellow mustard, wine, carp, celery, horse bean, jellyfish skin, Job's-tears, hyacinth bean, oregano, sweet basil, adzuki bean, bamboo shoot, soybean sprouts, and rosin

EDEMA

1. Wind-water syndrome ( )

Symptoms:
Cold or hot symptoms (3)
Cough (3)
Discharge of scant urine (4)*
Puffiness of eyelids or face, gradually extending towards the four limbs and the whole body at relatively high rate (6)*
Soreness in the joints with heavy sensations (4)*
Treatment principle: to expel wind and promote water flow
Treatment formula: *Yue-Bi-Jia-Zhu-Tang*
Food cures: carp, celery, horse bean, jellyfish skin, Job's-tears, prickly ash, hyacinth bean, oregano, sweet basil, bamboo shoot, soybean sprouts, rosin, adzuki bean, ambergris, barley, common carp, cucumber, mung bean, seaweed, shepherd's purse, star fruit, peppermint, spearmint, coconut meat, and green onion

2. Stoppage of internal water syndrome ( )

Symptoms:
Chest congestion (1)
Cold sensations in the back (1)
Deep and wiry pulse (1)
Dizziness (1)

Edema in the face (1)
Edema that fails to recover after being depressed by finger pressure (5)*
Intestinal rumbling (1)
Pain in the upper abdomen (1)
Pain induced by cough or spitting (1)
Severe edema in the limbs (6)*
Vomiting of bubbles (1)
Water noise in the stomach (1)
White and greasy coating on tongue (1)
Wiry pulse (1)
Treatment principle: to increase energy and promote water flow
Treatment formula: *Wu-Ling-San* or *Wu-Pi-Yin*
Food cures: adzuki bean, ambergris, barley, bamboo shoot, common carp, cucumber, mung bean, seaweed, shepherd's purse, and star fruit

3. Flooding of water-dampness syndrome ( )

Symptoms:
Ascites (1)
Diminished urination (2)
Chest congestion (1)
Difficult bowel movements (2)
Heavy sensations in the body (2)
Edema all over the body (9)*
Light edema in the eye socket as if just getting up from bed (1)
Thirst (2)
Treatment principle: to remove water drastically
Treatment formula: *Shu-Zao-Yin-Zi*
Food cures: carp, celery, horse bean, jellyfish skin, Job's-tears, prickly ash, hyacinth bean, oregano, sweet basil, bamboo shoot, soybean sprouts, rosin, adzuki bean, ambergris, barley, common carp, cucumber, mung bean, seaweed, shepherd's purse, and star fruit

4. Spleen yang deficiency syndrome ( )

Symptoms:
Abdominal pain (2)
Cold in the forehead that does not warm up (1)
Diarrhea (2)
Dysentery (2)
Edema that appears most severe in the lower half of the body (5)*
Edema that fails to return after being depressed by finger pressure (5)*
Stomachache (2)
Treatment principle: to warm and mobilize the spleen yang and to transform dampness and promote water flow
Treatment formula: *Shi-Pi-Yin*
Food cures: air bladder of shark, chicken, cayenne pepper, fennel, nutmeg, black and white pepper, prickly ash, mutton, sword bean, and white or yellow mustard

5. Kidneys yang deficiency syndrome ( )

Symptoms:
Cold feet, cold loins and legs, cold sensations in the genitals, or cold sensations in the muscles (1)
Cough and panting (1)
Diarrhea before dawn (1)
Diarrhea with sticky, muddy stools (1)
Discharge of watery, thin stools (1)
Dizziness (1)
Edema that appears most severe in the lower half of the body (3)*
Edema that fails to return after being depressed by finger pressure (2)*
Fatigue (1)
Frequent urination at night (1)
Lack of appetite (1)
Pain in the loins (lumbago)
Palpitations (1)
Panting (1)
Perspiration on the forehead (1)
Ringing in ears (1)
Wheezing (1)
Treatment principle: to warm the kidneys yang and promote water flow
Treatment formula: *Shen-Qi-Wan* or *Zhen-Wu-Tang*
Food cures: kidney, lobster, sardine, shrimp, sparrow, clove, dill seed, fennel, pistachio nut, sparrow egg, crab apple, raspberry, and walnut

DIMINISHED URINATION

1. Hot lungs syndrome ( )

Symptoms:
Acute panting in high-pitched sound with rapid expiration (1)
Bitter taste in the mouth (1)
Coughing out and vomiting of pus and blood with a fishy smell (1)
Coughing out yellow, sticky sputum (1)
Discharge of dry stools (1)
Discharge of yellow, sticky sputum in lumps (1)
Dripping of urine with difficult urination (2)*
Dry sensations in the mouth (1)
Flickering of nostrils (1)
Hot sensations in the body (1)
Light but periodic fever not unlike the tide (1)
Nosebleed (1)
Pain in the chest (1)
Pain in the throat (1)
Pain in throat with dry sensations and exhaling hot air from nose (1)
Paralysis (1)
Presence of sputum that can't be coughed out easily (1)

Psychological depression (1)
Throat swelling and red (1)
Urgent panting (1)

Treatment principle: to clear the heat in the lungs

Treatment formula: *Huang-Qin-Qing-Fei-Yin*

Food cures: apple, apple cucumber, apricot, white fungus, ham, jackfruit, lemon, maltose, mandarin orange, mulberry, olive, peach, pear, sweet potato, red and black date, tomato, white sugar, mung bean, and eggplant

2. Heart-fire syndrome ( )

Symptoms:
Bleeding from gums (1)
Cold hands and feet (1)
Difficult urination with reddish or very yellowish urine (3)*
Discharge of blood from the mouth (2)
Dribbling after urination (1)
Feeling miserable (1)
Hot sensations in the middle of palms (1)
Mouth canker (2)
Not alert (1)
Pain on urination (1)
Palpitations (2)
Pulpy and decayed tongue and mouth (1)
Seminal emission (1)
Sleeplessness (2)
Thirst (1)

Treatment principle: to clear the heat in the heart and sedate the fire

Treatment formula: *Dao-Chi-San*

Food cures: asparagus, pear peel, banana, bitter endive, black fungus, salt, spinach, strawberry, bamboo shoot, cucumber, Job's-tears, liver, leaf beet, mung bean,

peppermint, purslane, lily flower, salt, and cattail

3. Superficial dampness-heat syndrome ( )

Symptoms:
Burning sensation and itch in the genitals or burning sensation in the anus (1)
Burning sensation on urination (2)*
Diarrhea with forceful discharge of stools (1)
Discharge of yellowish-red, turbid stools with bad smell (1)
Edema (1)
Excessive perspiration (1)
Feeling miserable (1)
Frequent itch and pain in the vulva (1)
Jaundice (1)
Low fever (1)
Pain in the joints of the four limbs, with swelling and heaviness (1)
Paralysis (1)
Perspiration on hands and feet or the head (1)
Reddish and scant urine (1)
Retention of urine (1)
Scant, turbid urine (1)
Short streams of reddish urine (1)
Swollen body of the tongue (1)
Thirst (1)

Treatment principle: to clear the heat and remove the dampness and to promote urination

Treatment formula: *Jia-Wei-Si-Ling-San*

Food cures: carp, celery, horse bean, jellyfish skin, Job's-tears, prickly ash, hyacinth bean, oregano, sweet basil, adzuki bean, bamboo shoot, soybean sprouts, rosin, banana, bitter endive, black fungus, salt, spinach, strawberry, cucumber, leaf beet, mung bean, peppermint, and purslane

4. Energy deficiency syndrome ( )

Symptoms:
Abdominal pain (1)
Constipation with discharge of soft stools (1)
Discharge of sticky, turbid stools or diarrhea (1)
Dizziness (1)
Fatigued following bowel movement (1)
Headache (severe) that occurs with fatigue after labor (1)
Headache at intervals, headache in the morning, or prolonged headache (1)
Lying down with an inability to sit up, which will cause dizziness (1)
Misty vision (1)
Numbness (1)
Palpitations with insecure feeling (1)
Perspiration on hands and feet (1)
Prolonged headache (1)
Ringing in ears that causes deafness (1)
Shaking of hands (1)
Shortness of breath (1)
Swallowing difficulty (1)
Talking in weak voice (1)
Tips of four limbs slightly cold (1)
Underweight with dry skin (1)
Treatment principle: to strengthen energy and elevate the yang
Treatment formula: *Bu-Zhong-Yi-Qi-Tang*
Food cures: grape, longan nuts, maltose, mandarin fish, Irish potato, sweet rice, apple cucumber, bog bean, gold carp, carrot, chestnut, ham, horse bean, hyacinth bean, Job's-tears, royal jelly, string bean, whitefish, yam, red and black date, mutton, squash, and rock sugar

5. Excessive heat in the bladder syndrome ( )

Symptoms:
Discharge of urine containing pus and blood (3)
Hot pain inside the genitals on passing urine (3)
Muddy, unclear urine (2)
Obstructed and diminished urination in short streams (3)
Pain in lower abdomen with swollen feeling that is hard and full (3)
Urinary gravel (3)
Yellowish-red urine (3)
Treatment principle: to remove the heat from the bladder and promote urination
Treatment formula: *Tong-Guan-Wan*
Food cures: flour, duck, kelp, water spinach, banana, bitter endive, black fungus, salt, spinach, strawberry, bamboo shoot, cucumber, Job's-tears, leaf beet, mung bean, peppermint, and purslane

6. Blood coagulations syndrome ( )

Symptoms:
Abdominal pain (1)
Bleeding from gums (1)
Chest pain (1)
Coughing out blood (1)
Headache (1)
Jaundice (1)
Lumbago (1)
Pain (acute) around umbilicus resisting massage, and hard spots felt by hands (1)
Pain in region between navel and pubic hair with feeling of hardness (1)

Pain in the upper abdomen (1)
Pain in the loins as if being pierced with an awl (2)
Pain in the ribs (1)
Palpitations with insecure feeling (1)
Partial suppression of lochia (1)
Spasm (1)
Stomachache (1)
Stroke (1)
Swelling and congestion after eating (1)
Vomiting of blood (1)
Treatment principle: to break up the blood and remove coagulations
Treatment formula: *Dai-Di-Dang-Wan*
Food cures: ambergris, brown sugar, chestnut, eggplant, peach, black soybean, sturgeon, sweet basil, crab, distillers' grains, papaya, and saffron

7. Kidneys yang deficiency syndrome ( )

Symptoms:
Chronic diarrhea (1)
Cold feet, cold loins and legs, cold sensations in the genitals, or cold sensations in the muscles (1)
Cough and panting (1)
Diarrhea before dawn (1)
Diarrhea with sticky, muddy stools (1)
Discharge of water, thin stools (1)
Dizziness (1)
Edema (1)
Fatigue (1)
Frequent urination at night (1)
Hands and feet not warm (1)
Impotence (1)
Infertility (1)
Lack of appetite (1)
Pain in the loins (lumbago) (1)
Palpitations (1)
Panting (1)
Perspiration on the forehead (1)

Ringing in ears (1)
Scant urine (1)
Treatment principle: to warm and tone the kidneys yang
Treatment formula: *Shen-Qi-Wan*
Food cures: kidney, lobster, sardine, shrimp, sparrow, clove, dill seed, fennel, pistachio nut, sparrow egg, crab apple, raspberry, and walnut

INCONTINENCE OF URINATION

1. Spleen-lungs energy deficiency syndrome ( )

Symptoms:
Abdominal swelling (1)
Coughing out and spitting of sputum and saliva (1)
Decreased appetite (1)
Diarrhea with sticky, muddy stools (1)
Discharge of copious, clear, watery sputum (1)
Eating only a little with indigestion (1)
Fatigue of the four limbs (1)
Fatigue with lack of power (1)
Frequent desire to pass urine (4)*
Prolonged cough (1)
Rapid panting (1)
Shortness of breath (1)
Underweight (1)
Urine dribbling (4)*
Treatment principle: to strengthen energy and elevate the yang
Treatment formula: *Bu-Zhong-Yi-Qi-Tang*
Food cures: grape, longan nuts, maltose, mandarin fish, Irish potato, sweet rice, apple cucumber, bog bean, gold carp, carrot, chestnut, ham, horse bean, hyacinth bean, Job's-tears, royal jelly, string bean, whitefish, yam,

red and black date, mutton, squash, rock sugar, chicken egg yolk, and cheese

2. Kidneys energy deficiency syndrome (   )

Symptoms:
Deafness (2)
Dizziness (1)
Dribbling after urination (4)*
Fatigue (1)
Frequent urination with scant streams (4)*
Headache (1)
Impotence (2)
Lumbago (2)
Prolonged dizziness (1)
Ringing in ears (1)
Seminal emission (1)
Treatment principle: to warm and strengthen the kidneys and control urination
Treatment formula: *Suo-Niao-Wan* or *Shen-Qi-Wan*
Food cures: milk, millet, stamens, sword bean, wheat, black sesame seed, beef kidney, chestnut, chicken liver, lobster, perch, pork kidney, raspberry, sea cucumber, string bean, and walnut

3. Looseness of kidneys energy syndrome (   )

Symptoms:
Bed-wetting (5)*
Clear and long streams of urine (1)
Dizziness (1)
Dribbling of urine (1)
Fatigue (1)
Frequent urination particularly at night (1)
Incontinence of urination (1)
Pain and softness in the loins and the knees (1)

Premature ejaculation (1)
Ringing in ears (1)
Seminal emission (2)
Seminal emission without erotic dreams (2)
Vaginal discharge or bleeding (2)
Treatment principle: to strengthen energy and reinforce the kidneys
Treatment formula: *Sang-Piao-Xiao-San*
Food cures: gorgan fruit, chicken, walnuts, stamens, crab apple, yam, raspberry, and strawberry

SEMINAL EMISSION AND PREMATURE EJACULATION IN MEN

1. Deficiency fire syndrome (   )

Symptoms:
Coughing out blood (2)
Dry cough without sputum or coughing out slightly sticky fluids (1)
Dry sensations in the mouth (1)
Dry throat (1)
Feeling miserable (1)
Forgetfulness (1)
Hot sensations in body (1)
Illness attacks slowly but with a longer duration (chronic illness) (1)
Light but periodic fever not unlike the tide (1)
Night sweats (1)
Pain in the throat (1)
Ringing in ears (1)
Seminal emission with erotic dreams (2)*
Sleeplessness (1)
Sore loins (1)
Sputum with blood (1)
Toothache (2)
Treatment principle: to water the yin and sedate fire and to secure the heart and control emission

Treatment formula: *Feng-Sui-Dan* or *Zhi-Bai-Di-Huang-Wan*

Food cures: banana, bitter endive, black fungus, salt, spinach, strawberry, bamboo shoot, cucumber, Job's-tears, liver, leaf beet, mung bean, peppermint, purslane, lily flower, salt, cattail, chicken egg, duck egg, asparagus, royal jelly, pork, and oyster

2. Superficial dampness-heat syndrome (   )

Symptoms:

Abdominal pain (1)

Burning sensation and itch in the genitals or burning sensation in the anus (1)

Congested chest (1)

Diarrhea with forceful discharge of stool (1)

Discharge of yellowish-red, turbid stools with bad smell (1)

Edema (1)

Ejaculates running out along with urine (2)*

Excessive perspiration (1)

Jaundice (1)

Low fever (1)

Pain in the joints of the four limbs, with swelling and heaviness (1)

Pain inside the penis (2)*

Perspiration on hands and feet or the head (1)

Reddish and scant urine (1)

Retention of urine (1)

Seminal emission that occurs very frequently (2)*

Thirst (1)

Treatment principle: to clear dampness-heat and reinforce the kidneys energy to control semen

Treatment formula: *Bei-Xie-Fen-Qing-Yin*

Food cures: carp, celery, horse bean, jellyfish skin, Job's-tears, prickly ash, hyacinth bean, oregano, sweet basil, adzuki bean, bamboo shoot, soybean sprouts, rosin, banana, bitter endive, black fungus, salt, spinach, strawberry, cucumber, leaf beet, mung bean, peppermint, and purslane

3. Kidneys yin deficiency syndrome (   )

Symptoms:

Cold hands and feet (1)

Cough with sputum containing blood or coughing out fresh blood (1)

Deafness (1)

Dizziness (1)

Dry sensations in the mouth or dry throat (1)

Fatigue (1)

Feeling miserable and hurried, with fever (1)

Fever at night with burning sensations in internal organs (1)

Hot sensations in any part of the body (1)

Night sweats (1)

Pain in the heels (1)

Pain in the loins (lumbago) (1)

Pain in the tibia (1)

Ringing in ears (1)

Seminal emission mostly without dreams (1)*

Sleeplessness (1)

Sore loins and weak legs (1)

Spots in front of the eyes (1)

Thirst (1)

Toothache or loose teeth (1)

Treatment principle: to strengthen the kidneys yin to control ejaculation

Treatment formula: *Liu-Wei-Di-Huang-Wan* or *Zuo-Gui-Wan*

Food cures: abalone, asparagus, chicken egg, cuttlefish, duck, duck egg, white fungus, oyster, pork, royal jelly, chestnut, chicken liver, and pork kidneys

4. Kidneys energy deficiency syndrome ( )

Symptoms:
Cold sensations in the genitals (3)*
Deafness (2)
Dizziness (2)
Fatigue (2)
Headache (2)
Impotence (2)
Lumbago (2)
Prolonged dizziness (1)
Ringing in ears (2)
Seminal emission that occurs spontaneously as if semen were just sliding out (2)*
Treatment principle: to tone the kidneys energy and control the semen gate
Treatment formula: *You-Gui-Wan* or *Jin-Suo-Gu-Jing-Wan*
Food cures: milk, millet, stamens, sword bean, wheat, black sesame seed, beef kidney, chestnut, chicken liver, lobster, perch, pork kidney, raspberry, sea cucumber, string bean, and walnut

IMPOTENCE IN MEN

1. Deficiency fire syndrome ( )

Symptoms:
Coughing out blood (1)
Dry cough without sputum or coughing out slightly sticky fluids (1)
Dry sensations in the mouth or dry throat (1)
Feeling miserable (1)
Forgetfulness (1)
Hot sensations in body (1)

Illness attacks slowly but with a longer duration (chronic illness)
Light but periodic fever not unlike the tide (1)
Night sweats (1)
Pain in the throat (1)
Ringing in ears (1)
Seminal emission with dreams (1)
Sleeplessness (1)
Sore loins (1)
Sputum with blood (1)
Strong sexual desire with very quick ejaculation (5)*
Toothache (1)
Treatment principle: to sedate fire and tone the kidneys yin
Treatment formula: *Zhi-Bai-Di-Huang-Wan*
Food cures: banana, bitter endive, black fungus, salt, spinach, strawberry, bamboo shoot, cucumber, Job's-tears, liver, leaf beet, mung bean, peppermint, purslane, lily flower, salt, cattail, chicken egg, duck egg, asparagus, royal jelly, pork, and oyster

2. Spleen deficiency syndrome ( )

Symptoms:
Chronic diarrhea (2)
Chronic dysentery (2)
Lack of firm erection (6)*
Poor appetite (1)
Prolapse of any internal organ (6)*
Prolapse of anus (2)
Shortness of breath (1)
Treatment principle: to tone energy and strengthen the spleen
Treatment formula: *Bu-Zhong-Yi-Qi-Tang*
Food cures: longan nuts, mandarin fish, apple cucumber, gold carp, carrot, chestnut, corncob, Job's-tears, Irish potato, rice, royal jelly,

string bean, yam, beef, and red and black date

3. Kidneys yang deficiency syndrome ( )

Symptoms:
Cold feet, cold loins and legs, or cold sensations in the genitals (1)
Diarrhea before dawn (2)
Diarrhea with sticky, muddy stools (1)
Dizziness (1)
Edema (2)
Excessive perspiration (1)
Fatigue (2)
Frequent urination at night (1)
Panting (2)
Perspiration on the forehead (1)
Retention of urine (1)
Ringing in ears (1)
Scant urine (1)
Seminal emission (2)
Shortness of breath (1)
Treatment principle: to warm the kidneys and reinforce kidneys yang energy
Treatment formula: *You-Gui-Wan*
Food cures: kidney, lobster, sardine, shrimp, sparrow, clove, dill seed, fennel, pistachio nut, sparrow egg, crab apple, raspberry, and walnuts

INFERTILITY IN WOMEN

1. Simultaneous deficiency of energy and blood syndrome ( )

Symptoms:
Bleeding of various kinds with blood in light color, often seen in consumptive diseases (1)
Dizziness (1)
Fatigue (1)
Flying objects seen in front of the eyes (1)

Insomnia (1)
Irregular menstruation (1)
Low energy (1)
Low voice (1)
Menstrual flow in light-red color (4)*
Mentally depressed (1)
Regular menstruation, but with very scant flow, lasting for one or two days only (3)*
Numbness of limbs (1)
Pale complexion and lips (1)
Pale nails (1)
Palpitations (1)
Treatment principle: to tone the energy and the blood simultaneously and to tone the kidneys
Treatment formula: *Ba-Zhen-Yi-Mu-Wan*
Food cures: abalone, asparagus, cuttlefish, chicken egg, duck egg, white fungus, beef liver, grape, mandarin fish, oyster, milk, beef, cherry, blood clam, longan nuts, maltose, Irish potato, sweet rice, apple cucumber, bog bean, gold carp, carrot, chestnut, ham, horse bean, hyacinth bean, Job's-tears, royal jelly, string bean, whitefish, yam, red and black date, mutton, squash, and rock sugar

2. Yin deficiency syndrome ( )

Symptoms:
Bleeding from gums (1)
Constipation (1)
Dizziness (1)
Dry and scant stools, dry sensations in the mouth, or dry throat (1)
Fatigue (1)
Headache in the afternoon (1)
Low fever in the afternoon (1)
Menstrual flow in dark color (1)*
Night sweats (1)

Nosebleed (1)

Pain in the throat, also red and swollen (1)

Palms of hands and soles of feet are both hot (1)

Palpitations with insecure feeling (1)

Regular menstruation with scant flow, lasting for half day or one day (1)*

Short and reddish streams of urine (1)

Sleeplessness (1)

Swallowing difficulty (1)

Toothache (1)

Underweight (1)

Vomiting of blood or nosebleed during menstrual periods (1)

Treatment principle: to water the yin and clear the heat and to nourish the blood and regulate menstruation

Treatment formula: *Yang-Jing-Zhong-Yu-Tang, Qing-Gu-Zi-Shen-Tang,* or *Qing-Xue-Yang-Yin-Tang*

Food cures: bird's nest, cheese, kidney bean, abalone, asparagus, chicken egg, cuttlefish, duck, duck egg, white fungus, oyster, pork, and royal jelly

3. Cold and deficient womb syndrome ( )

Symptoms:

Cold pain or cold sensations in the lower abdomen or cold sensations in the genitals (10)*

Dark, blackish menstrual flow (1)

Failure of the fetus to grow (1)

Fetus motion (1)

Frequent miscarriage (1)

Functional disturbances of the ovary (1)

Habitual miscarriage (1)

Pale complexion (1)

Poor appetite (1)

Thin and watery menstrual flow in light color (1)

Underdevelopment of the womb (1)

Treatment principle: to warm the womb

Treatment formula: *Ai-Fu-Nuan-Gong-Wan*

Food cures: cinnamon, kidneys, lobster, sheep's milk, sardine, shrimp, star anise, red and black date, and sword bean

4. Hot blood syndrome ( )

Symptoms:

Abdominal pain that occurs at onset of menstrual periods (1)

Deep-red or violet menstrual flow (1)

Discharge of blood from anus before periods (1)

Fever after childbirth (1)

Irregularity of menstrual periods (1)

Menstrual flow somewhat heavy (1)

Menstrual flow with a bad smell (1)

Nosebleed (1)

Plentiful menstrual flow (1)

Premature menstrual periods, which may be more than 10 days early or two periods within one month (7)*

Red and plentiful menstrual flow (1)

Skin ulcers (1)

Vaginal bleeding (1)

Vomiting of blood or nosebleed during menstrual periods (1)

Treatment principle: to clear the heat in the blood

Treatment formula: *Qing-Jing-Tang*

Food cures: bitter endive, camellia, cattail, black fungus, salt, spinach, strawberry, banana, cucumber, and licorice

5. Liver energy congestion syndrome ( )

Symptoms:

Abdominal pain (1)

Convulsions (1)
Irregularity of menstrual periods (1)
Menstrual pain (5)*
Morning sickness (1)
Numbness (1)
Pain in the upper abdomen (2)
Premature periods or overdue periods (1)
Shortage of milk secretion after childbirth (1)
Stomachache (2)
Subjective sensations of objects in the throat (2)
Vomiting of blood (1)
Whitish vaginal discharge (1)
Treatment principle: to relax the liver and disperse energy congestion
Treatment formula: *Xiao-Yao-San* or *De-Sheng-Dan*
Food cures: brown sugar, garlic, turmeric, kumquat, beef, cherry, bird's nest, butterfish, chicken, coconut meat, date, tofu, mustard seed, sweet rice, goose meat, mutton, jackfruit, squash, sweet potato, red and black date, rice, rock sugar, caraway seed, spearmint, common button mushroom, oregano, red bean, ambergris, dill seed, garlic, sweet basil, and saffron

6. Dampness-sputum syndrome ( )

Symptoms:
Discharge of sputum that can be coughed out easily or discharge of white, watery sputum (1)
Dizziness (1)
Excessive whitish vaginal discharge (1)
Frequent coughs during pregnancy that are prolonged and cause motion of fetus (1)

Headache (1)
Hiccups (1)
Light-red menstrual flow (1)
Menstrual periods overdue frequently (1)
Morning sickness (1)
Turbid and sticky menstrual flow (1)
Pain in the chest (1)
Panting (1)
Plentiful menstrual flow (1)
Prolonged dizziness (1)
Sleep a lot or sleeplessness (1)
Susceptible to morning sickness during pregnancy (1)
Suppression of menses (1)
Vomiting (1)
White, sliding sputum that can be cleared from throat easily (1)
Whitish vaginal discharge (1)
Treatment principle: to strengthen the spleen and dry up dampness
Treatment formula: *Qi-Gong-Wan*
Food cures: adzuki bean, ambergris, barley, common carp, cucumber, mung bean, seaweed, shepherd's purse, star fruit, bamboo shoot, crown daisy, date, fresh ginger, leaf or brown mustard, black and white pepper, white or yellow mustard seed, asparagus, and pear

SLEEPINESS, INCLUDING DROWSINESS, LETHARGY, AND NARCOLEPSY

1. Spleen-dampness syndrome ( )

Symptoms:
Chest discomfort without appetite (1)
Diarrhea (1)
Edema (1)
Feeling sleepy all day long (4)*
Heavy sensations in head as if the head were covered with something (1)

Heavy sensations in the body with a
    desire to lie down (5)*
Jaundice (1)
Love of hot drink (1)
Nausea and vomiting (1)
Plentiful vaginal discharge (1)
Stomach fullness and discomfort (1)
Sweet, sticky taste in mouth (1)
Too tired to talk or move (1)
Treatment principle: to dry up
    dampness, strengthen the spleen,
    and wake up the spirits
Treatment formula: *Tai-Wu-Shen-
    Zhu-San, Hou-Pu-Xia-Ling-Tang,
    Wei-Ling-Tang,* or *San-Ren-Tang*
Food cures: gold carp, corncob,
    horse bean, Job's-tears, prickly
    ash, adzuki bean, and bamboo
    shoot

2. Dampness-sputum syndrome (   )

Symptoms:
Cough (1)
Discharge of sputum that can be
    coughed out easily (1)
Discharge of white, watery sputum
    (1)
Dizziness (1)
Excessive whitish vaginal discharge
    (1)
Frequent coughs during pregnancy
    that are prolonged and cause
    motion of fetus (1)
Headache (1)
Hiccups (1)
Pain in the chest (1)
Panting (2)
Prolonged dizziness (1)
Sleep a lot (3)*
Sleeplessness (1)
Suppression of menses (1)
Vomiting (2)
White, sliding sputum that can be
    cleared from throat easily (1)

Treatment principle: to transform
    sputum and wake up the spirits
Treatment formula: *Wen-Dan-Tang*
Food cures: adzuki bean, ambergris,
    barley, common carp, cucumber,
    mung bean, seaweed, shepherd's
    purse, star fruit, bamboo shoot,
    crown daisy, date, fresh ginger,
    leaf or brown mustard, black and
    white pepper, white or yellow
    mustard seed, asparagus, and pear

3. Spleen energy deficiency syndrome (   )

Symptoms:
Abdominal pain (2)
Diarrhea (2)
Edema (1)
Fatigue (3)*
Feeling sleepy particularly after meals
    (4)*
Lips rolled up (1)
Loud snoring during sleep (3)*
Stiff tongue (1)
Stomachache (2)
Vomiting of blood (1)
Treatment principle: to strengthen
    the spleen and energy
Treatment formula: *Xiang-Sha-Liu-
    Jun-Zi-Tang* or *Cang-Er-Zi-San* with
    Er-Chen-Tang
Food cures: grape, longan nuts,
    maltose, mandarin fish, Irish
    potato, sweet rice, apple
    cucumber, bog bean, gold carp,
    carrot, chestnut, ham, horse bean,
    hyacinth bean, Job's-tears, royal
    jelly, string bean, whitefish, yam,
    red and black date, mutton,
    squash, rock sugar, and chicken
    egg yolk

4. Yang deficiency syndrome (   )

Symptoms:
Clear and long streams of urine (1)

Cold hands and feet (1)
Constipation (1)
Diarrhea (1)
Diminished urination (1)
Discharge of watery, thin stools (1)
Edema (1)
Fatigue (1)
Fear of cold (1)
Fingertips often cold (1)
Forgetfulness (1)
Frequent fear of cold in hands and feet (1)
Headache in the morning (1)
Older patients (2)*
Palpitations (1)
Perspiration due to hot weather or putting on warm clothes (1)
Perspiration like cold water (1)
Scant energy and too tired to talk (1)
Sleep a lot (1)
Treatment principle: to strengthen energy and warm the yang
Treatment formula: *Fu-Zi-Li-Zhong-Wan* with *Shen-Qi-Wan*
Food cures: kidneys, lobster, sardine, shrimp, star anise, and red and black date

5. Blood coagulations syndrome ( )

Symptoms:
Abdominal pain (1)
Chest pain (1)
Coughing out blood (1)
Headache (1)
History of past injuries (2)*
Jaundice (1)
Lumbago (1)
Pain in the upper abdomen (1)
Pain in the loins as if being pierced with an awl (1)
Palpitations with insecure feeling (1)
Sleep for about 10 minutes each time (2)*
Spasm (1)

Stomachache
Symptoms worsening in the afternoon and at night (2)*
Vomiting of blood (1)
Treatment principle: to activate the blood and remove blood coagulations
Treatment formula: *Tong-Qiao-Huo-Xue-Tang* or *Fu-Yuan-Huo-Xue-Tang*
Food cures: ambergris, brown sugar, chestnut, eggplant, peach, black soybean, sturgeon, sweet basil, crab, distillers' grains, papaya, and saffron

6. Liver energy congestion syndrome ( )

Symptoms:
Abdominal obstruction (2)
Abdominal pain (2)
Bitter taste in the mouth (3)*
Convulsions (1)
Dizziness (1)
Numbness (1)
Pain in the upper abdomen (2)
Sleep a lot normally (3)*
Stomachache (2)
Subjective sensations of objects in the throat (2)
Vomiting of blood (1)
Treatment principle: to disperse liver energy congestion
Treatment formula: *Dan-Zhi-Xiao-Yao-San*
Food cures: brown sugar, garlic, turmeric, kumquat, beef, cherry, bird's nest, butterfish, chicken, coconut meat, date, tofu, mustard seed, sweet rice, goose meat, mutton, jackfruit, squash, sweet potato, red and black date, rice, rock sugar, caraway seed, spearmint, common button mushroom, oregano, red bean, ambergris, dill seed, sweet basil, and saffron

7. Heart energy deficiency syndrome ( )

Symptoms:
Chest pain (2)
Epilepsy (2)
Fatigue (2)
Forgetfulness (2)
Insomnia (2)
Nervousness (2)
Pain in the heart (2)
Palpitations (2)
Spells of sleep mostly (3)*
White complexion (1)
Treatment principle: to strengthen heart energy and secure the spirits
Treatment formula: *Yang-Xin-Tang*
Food cures: air bladder of shark, water spinach, abalone, asparagus, dried ginger, and cinnamon

OBESITY

1. Spleen-dampness syndrome ( )

Symptoms:
Chest discomfort without appetite (1)
Diarrhea (1)
Edema (3)*
Heavy sensations in head as if the head were covered with something (1)
Heavy sensations in the body with discomfort (1)
Jaundice (1)
Love of hot drink (1)
Nausea and vomiting (1)
Poor appetite (4)*
Scant urine (3)*
Stomach fullness and discomfort (1)
Sweet, sticky taste in mouth (1)
Too tired to talk or move (1)
Treatment principle: to strengthen the spleen and remove dampness
Treatment formula: *Fang-Ji-Huang-Qi-Tang* with *Ling-Gui-Zhu-Gan-Tang*

Food cures: gold carp, corncob, horse bean, Job's-tears, prickly ash, adzuki bean, and bamboo shoot

2. Spleen and stomach heat and dampness syndrome ( )

Symptoms:
Abdominal swelling (1)*
Bad breath (1)
Bleeding from gums (1)
Dizziness (1)*
Constipation (1)*
Foul breath from the mouth (1)
Getting hungry easily (1)
Gums swelling (1)
Hiccups (1)
Light taste in the mouth (1)
Nosebleed (1)
Pain in the gums with swelling (1)
Pain in the throat (1)
Perspiring on the head (1)
Stomachache (1)
Thirst and craving for cold (1)
Vomiting (1)
Vomiting of blood (1)
Vomiting right after eating (1)
Vomiting with stomach discomfort as if hungry, empty, or hot (1)
Treatment principle: to clear the heat in the stomach and remove dampness from the stomach
Treatment formula: *Fang-Feng-Tong-Sheng-San*
Food cures: carp, celery, horse bean, jellyfish skin, Job's-tears, prickly ash, hyacinth bean, oregano, sweet basil, adzuki bean, bamboo shoot, soybean sprouts, rosin, banana, bitter endive, black fungus, salt, spinach, strawberry, cucumber, leaf beet, mung bean, peppermint, and purslane

3. Liver energy congestion syndrome ( )

Symptoms:
Abdominal obstruction (2)
Abdominal pain (2)
Bitter taste in the mouth (3)*
Convulsions (1)
Dry tongue (1)
Getting angry easily (3)*
Numbness (1)
Pain in the upper abdomen (2)
Poor appetite (2)*
Stomachache (2)
Subjective sensations of objects in the throat (2)
Vomiting of blood (1)
Treatment principle: to disperse liver energy congestion
Treatment formula: *Da-Chai-Hu-Tang*
Food cures: brown sugar, garlic, turmeric, kumquat, beef, cherry, bird's nest, butterfish, chicken, coconut meat, date, tofu, mustard seed, sweet rice, goose meat, mutton, jackfruit, squash, sweet potato, red and black date, rice, rock sugar, caraway seed, spearmint, common button mushroom, oregano, red bean, ambergris, dill seed, sweet basil, and saffron

4. Simultaneous energy congestion and blood coagulations syndrome ( )

Symptoms:
Abdominal swelling (2)
Chronic hepatitis (1)
Cirrhosis (1)
Congested chest (1)
Irregular menstruation with blood clots in women (1)
Love of sighing (1)
Lump in the abdomen that stays in the same region (1)
Pain in the upper abdomen (4)*
Palpitations (4)*
Shortness of breath (4)*
Treatment principle: to regulate energy and remove blood coagulations
Treatment formula: *Tao-Hong-Si-Wu-Tang*
Food cures: beef, cherry, bird's nest, butterfish, chicken, coconut meat, date, tofu, mustard seed, sweet rice, goose meat, mutton, jackfruit, squash, sweet potato, red and black date, rice, rock sugar, caraway seed, spearmint, common button mushroom, oregano, red bean, ambergris, dill seed, garlic, sweet basil, saffron, ambergris, brown sugar, chestnut, eggplant, peach, black soybean, sturgeon, crab, distillers' grains, papaya, and saffron

5. Internal sputum syndrome ( )

Symptoms:
Abdominal swelling or rumbling (1)
Congested chest (1)
Dizziness (3)*
Headache (1)
Heaviness in the body (3)*
Love of hot drink (1)
Love of sweet or greasy foods (2)*
Numbness (2)*
Pain in the chest or upper abdomen (1)
Palpitations (1)
Stomachache (1)
Swollen body of the tongue (1)
Vomiting or coughing out watery sputum in large amounts (2)*
Treatment principle: to strengthen the spleen and transform sputum
Treatment formula: *Wen-Dan-Tang*
Food cures: bamboo shoot, crown daisy, date, fresh ginger, leaf or

brown mustard, mustard seed, black and white pepper, white or yellow mustard seed, asparagus, and pear

6. Spleen-kidneys yang deficiency syndrome (   )

Symptoms:
Abdominal swelling (1)
Cold hands and feet or cold loins (1)
Diarrhea before dawn (1)
Diarrhea with sticky, muddy stools (1)
Dysentery (1)
Eating very little (1)
Edema (1)
Edema that occurs all over the body (1)
Fatigue (1)
Fear of cold (1)
Four limbs weakness (1)
Frequent urination with clear or white urine (1)
Mentally fatigued (1)
Poor appetite (2)*
Scant urine (2)*
Sputum rumbling with panting (1)
Watery stools (2)*
Treatment principle: to warm the kidneys and strengthen the spleen
Treatment formula: *Zhen-Wu-Tang* with *Huang-Ji-Huang-Qi-Tang*
Food cures: air bladder of shark, chicken, cayenne pepper, fennel, nutmeg, black and white pepper, prickly ash, mutton, sword bean, white or yellow mustard, kidney, lobster, sardine, shrimp, sparrow, clove, dill seed, fennel, pistachio nut, sparrow egg, crab apple, raspberry, and walnut

3

TREATMENT OF
DIAGNOSED DISORDERS

HYPERTENSION AND HYPOTENSION

The normal blood pressure is the systolic pressure between 90 and 140 mm of mercury and the diastolic pressure between 60 and 90 mm of mercury. Hypertension means that the systolic pressure is over 140 and the diastolic pressure is over 90 mm of mercury. Hypotension means that the systolic pressure is lower than 90 and the diastolic pressure is lower than 60 mm of mercury.

Hypertension

1. Liver-fire syndrome (   )

Symptoms:
Bitter taste in the mouth (2)
Blood pressure rises readily with
    anger or stress (1)*
Discharge of yellowish and scant
    urine (2)
Dry mouth (2)
Hot temper (2)
Red eyes (2)
Red face (2)
Severe headache (2)
Vertigo (2)
Treatment principle: to reduce liver-fire and nourish the yin

Treatment formula: *Long-Dan-Xie-Gan-Tang*
Food cures: 1. Boil 100 g seaweed to eat every day; 2. wash and cut up 60 g celery to boil with 60 g rice for one-day consumption and continue for 10 days; 3. boil 30 g fresh water chestnut with 30 g jellyfish skin (with salt washed off) in water for consumption two times daily; 4. boil kelp and mung bean, 60 g each, until both are extremely soft, and then season with brown sugar to drink once daily for one week. Foods: spinach, chestnut, shepherd's purse, rye, black fungus, vinegar, abalone, asparagus, chicken egg, white fungus, pork, and royal jelly.

2. Liver and kidneys yin deficiency with liver yang upsurging syndrome (   )

Symptoms:
Blood pressure rises readily with
    fatigue and stress (4)
Discharge of reddish and scant urine
    (2)
Hot temper (1)
Insomnia (2)
Lumbago (2)
Many dreams (2)

107

Numbness of the four limbs (2)
Pain in the legs (2)
Ringing in the ears (2)
Seminal emission in men (2)
Vertigo (2)
Treatment principle: to nourish liver yin and kidney yin and to suppress liver yang
Treatment formula: *Zhen-Gan-Xi-Feng-Tang*
Food cures: 1. Prepare a pork gallbladder, squeeze as many black soybeans as possible into the gallbladder, steam it until cooked, and dry it under the sun; eat 20 to 30 black soybeans each time, twice daily, for one week. 2. Wash and soak 250 g fresh celery in hot water for 20 minutes, cut up the celery to squeeze juice, season with white sugar to drink like tea, once daily for a few days. Foods: bird's nest, cheese, chicken egg, kidney bean, brown sugar, mussel, abalone, asparagus, chicken egg, cuttlefish, duck, duck egg, white fungus, oyster, pork, royal jelly, chestnut, chicken liver, and pork kidneys.

3. Both yin and yang are deficient with deficient yang moving upward syndrome ( )

Symptoms:
Blurred vision (1)
Cold limbs (2)
Dry mouth (1)
Frequent urination at night (2)
Heavy breathing on walking (2)
Insomnia (1)
Light headache (1)
Lumbago (1)
Many dreams (1)
Perspiration (1)

Ringing in the ears (2)
Slightly red face (1)
Twitching of muscles (2)
Vertigo (1)
Weak legs (1)
Treatment principle: to tone both the yin and the yang
Treatment formula: *Shen-Qi-Wan*
Food cures: Boil 300 g fresh celery with five red dates until cooked; drink the soup and eat celery and dates once daily for one week. Foods: chicken egg yolk, cheese, kidney bean, abalone, cuttlefish, duck, duck egg, white fungus, oyster, pork, royal jelly, and celery.

Hypotension

1. Heart yang deficiency syndrome ( )

Symptoms:
Cold sensations (1)
Fatigue (1)
Getting scared easily with rapid heartbeats (1)
Female patient (3)*
Hands and feet extremely cold (1)
Over sixty years old (3)*
Pain in the chest (2)
Pain in the heart (2)
Palpitations with insecure feeling (1)
Perspiring heavily (1)
Systolic pressure below 90 mm of mercury (3)*
Unconsciousness (1)
Treatment principle: to tone the heart yang
Treatment formula: *Gui-Zhi-Gan-Cao-Tang*
Food cures: dried ginger, cinnamon, wheat, water spinach, kidneys, lobster, sardine, shrimp, star anise, and red and black date

2. Spleen-stomach yang deficiency syndrome ( )

Symptoms:
Abdominal pain (1)
Abdominal swelling after meals (2)*
Cold limbs (1)
Diarrhea (2)*
Fatigue (1)
Intermittent hiccups with low sound (1)
Love of warmth and massage (1)
Pain worsening with fatigue and hunger (1)
Pain improving with rest and eating (1)
Palpitations (2)*
Poor appetite (1)
Shortness of breath (1)
Stomachache (1)
Upset stomach (1)
Vomiting of undigested foods (2)
Water noise in the stomach (1)
Withered and yellowish complexion (1)

Treatment principle: to tone the spleen and the stomach and to increase blood and energy

Treatment formula: *Dang-Gui-Jian-Zhong-Tang*

Food cures: air bladder of shark, chicken, cayenne pepper, fennel, nutmeg, black and white pepper, prickly ash, mutton, sword bean, white or yellow mustard, cardamon seed, carp, cinnamon, garlic, and beef

3. Spleen-kidneys deficiency syndrome ( )

Symptoms:
Deafness (1)
Diarrhea (1)
Difficult urination (1)
Dizziness (9)*

Fatigue of the four limbs (1)
Forgetfulness (1)
Insomnia (1)
Misty vision (1)
Palpitations (1)
Ringing in the ears (1)
Shortness of breath (1)
Yellowish complexion (1)

Treatment principle: to tone the spleen and the kidneys

Treatment formula: *Shen-Huang-Gan-Qi-Tang*

Food cures: chicken egg yolk, common button mushroom, wheat bran, rice, beef, cherry, bird's nest, coconut meat, date, tofu, mustard seed, sweet potato, red and black date, rock sugar, apple cucumber, carrot, chestnut, Irish potato, abalone, asparagus, chicken egg, white fungus, black sesame seed, beef kidney, chicken liver, lobster, pork kidney, raspberry, scallop, sea cucumber, shrimp, string bean, and walnut

4. Simultaneous deficiency of yin and energy syndrome ( )

Symptoms:
Constipation (1)
Dizziness (1)
Dry cough with scant sputum (1)
Dry mouth (1)
Discharge of dry stools (1)
Excessive perspiration (2)
Fatigue (1)
Fever (1)
Frequent vomiting (1)
Hot sensations in the palms of hands and soles of feet (1)
Light stomachache with swelling (2)
Palpitations (2)
Poor appetite (1)
Scant urine (1)

Sore throat (1)
Thirst (1)
Too tired to talk (1)
Treatment principle: to tone the energy and the yin simultaneously
Treatment formula: *Sheng-Mai-San*
Food cures: bird's nest, cheese, kidney bean, abalone, asparagus, chicken egg, cuttlefish, duck, duck egg, white fungus, oyster, pork, royal jelly, grape, longan nuts, maltose, mandarin fish, Irish potato, sweet rice, apple cucumber, bog bean, gold carp, carrot, chestnut, ham, horse bean, hyacinth bean, Job's-tears, royal jelly, string bean, whitefish, yam, red and black date, mutton, squash, and rock sugar

5. Heart-kidneys yang deficiency syndrome (   )

Symptoms:
Cold limbs (1)
Cold sweats (1)
Discharge of watery, thin stools (1)
Edema (2)
Frequent urination particularly at night (1)
Heavy head with light feet sensations (4)*
Orthostatic hypotension (hypotension occurring when a person assumes an erect position) (3)*
Pain in the chest (2)
Palpitations (2)
Nervousness (2)
Shock (1)
Treatment principle: to tone the heart yang and the kidney yang
Treatment formula: *Shen-Fu-Tang*
Food cures: dried ginger, cinnamon, wheat, water spinach, kidneys, star anise, red and black date, lobster, sardine, shrimp, sparrow,

clove, dill seed, fennel, pistachio nut, sparrow egg, crab apple, raspberry, and walnut

HIGH CHOLESTEROL

1. Superficial dampness-heat syndrome (   )

Symptoms:
Abdominal swelling or pain (2)*
Burning sensation and itch in the genitals or burning sensation in the anus (1)
Congested chest (1)
Diarrhea with forceful discharge of stools (1)
Discharge of yellowish-red, turbid stools with bad smell (1)
Edema (2)*
Excessive perspiration (1)
Feeling miserable (1)
Itch and pain in the vulva frequently (1)
Jaundice (1)
Pain in the joints of the four limbs, with swelling and heaviness (1)
Perspiration on hands and feet or the head (1)
Reddish and scant urine, retention of urine, or short streams of reddish urine (1)
Swollen body of the tongue (1)
Thirst (1)
Yellowish body color (1)
Treatment principle: to clear heat and remove dampness
Treatment formula: *Xiao-Zhi-Tang*
Food cures: carp, celery, horse bean, jellyfish skin, Job's-tears, prickly ash, hyacinth bean, oregano, sweet basil, adzuki bean, bamboo shoot, soybean sprouts, rosin, banana, bitter endive, black fungus, salt, spinach, strawberry, cucumber, leaf beet, mung bean, peppermint, and purslane

2. Spleen-sputum syndrome ( )

Symptoms:
Abdominal swelling (1)
Abundant saliva (3)
Coughing out watery sputum (6)*
Fatigue (4)*
Overweight, but eat only a small amount of food (1)
Poor appetite (1)
Slight fullness of the stomach (2)
Suppression of menses (1)
Weakened limbs (1)
Treatment principle: to strengthen the spleen, harmonize the stomach, remove sputum, and transform dampness
Treatment formula: *Jia-Wei-Er-Chen-Tang*
Food cures: bamboo shoot, crown daisy, date, fresh ginger, leaf or brown mustard, black and white pepper, white or yellow mustard seed, asparagus, and pear

3. Hot stomach syndrome ( )

Symptoms:
Bad breath (1)
Bleeding from gums (1)
Foul breath from the mouth (1)
Getting hungry easily (1)
Gums swelling (1)
Hiccups (1)
Morning sickness (1)
Nosebleed (1)
Pain in the gums with swelling (2)
Pain in the throat (1)
Perspiring on the head (1)
Stomachache (2)
Thirst and craving for cold (1)
Vomiting (1)
Vomiting of blood (2)
Vomiting right after eating (1)
Vomiting with stomach discomfort as if hungry, empty, or hot (1)

Treatment principle: to clear the internal heat and promote bowel movements
Treatment formula: *Da-Cheng-Qi-Tang*
Food cures: salt, lily flower, bitter endive, camellia, cattail, black fungus, spinach, strawberry, banana, cucumber, and licorice

4. Liver-fire upsurging syndrome ( )

Symptoms:
Acute dizziness (1)
Bleeding from stomach (1)
Congested chest (1)
Deafness (1)
Dim eyes (1)
Dizziness (1)
Dry sensations in the mouth (1)
Feeling hurried and quick tempered or feeling insecure about sleep (1)
Getting angry easily (1)
Headache on both sides of the head and in the corners of the eyes (1)
Headache that is severe (1)
Hiccups (1)
Insanity (1)
Nosebleed (1)
Pain in the chest and the upper abdomen (1)
Red eyes (1)
Ringing in ears (1)
Sleeplessness or sleep a lot (1)
Vomiting of blood (1)
Yellowish-red urine (1)
Treatment principle: to clear the heat and sedate the fire in the liver
Treatment formula: *Long-Dan-Xie-Gan-Tang*
Food cures: spinach, chestnut, shepherd's purse, rye, black fungus, vinegar, abalone, asparagus, chicken egg, white fungus, pork, and royal jelly

5. Spleen-kidneys yang deficiency syndrome ( )

Symptoms:
Abdominal swelling (1)
Cold hands and feet or cold loins (1)
Diarrhea before dawn (1)
Diarrhea with sticky, muddy stools (1)
Eating only a little (1)
Edema (1)
Edema that occurs all over the body (1)
Fatigue (1)
Fear of cold (1)
Flying objects seen in front of the eyes (3)*
Four limbs weakness (1)
Frequent urination with clear or white urine (1)
Lumbago (1)
Mentally fatigued (1)
Over 65 years old (3)*
Sputum rumbling with panting (1)
Treatment principle: to tone the kidneys and the spleen yang
Treatment formula: *Qing-Zhi-Tang*
Food cures: air bladder of shark, chicken, cayenne pepper, fennel, nutmeg, black and white pepper, prickly ash, mutton, sword bean, white or yellow mustard, kidney, lobster, sardine, shrimp, sparrow, clove, dill seed, fennel, pistachio nut, sparrow egg, crab apple, raspberry, and walnuts

6. Simultaneous deficiency of energy and blood syndrome ( )

Symptoms:
Arteriosclerosis patient (2)*

Bleeding of various kinds with blood in light color, often seen in consumptive diseases (1)
Chest pain or congestion (2)*
Dizziness (2)
Fatigue (2)
Flying objects seen in front of the eyes (1)
Insomnia (2)
Low energy (1)
Low voice (1)
Numbness of limbs (1)
Pale complexion and lips (1)
Pale nails (1)
Palpitations (2)
Ringing in the ears (1)
Treatment principle: to regulate energy and activate the blood
Treatment formula: *Guan-Xin-Er-Hao-Fang*
Food cures: abalone, asparagus, cuttlefish, chicken egg, duck egg, white fungus, beef liver, grape, mandarin fish, oyster, milk, beef, cherry, blood clam, longan nuts, maltose, Irish potato, sweet rice, apple cucumber, bog bean, gold carp, carrot, chestnut, ham, horse bean, hyacinth bean, Job's-tears, royal jelly, string bean, whitefish, yam, red and black date, mutton, squash, and rock sugar
Research: Another formula called *Dan-Tian-Jiang-Zhi-Wan* has been found to lower cholesterol. According to a relatively recent research project involving 251 subjects with high cholesterol, after treatment with this formula 33 percent showed significant improvement. Take 4 grams of this herbal powder each day in two doses (one in the morning and one in the afternoon) for three months for best results.**

** Journal of Traditional Chinese Medicine, 1986:39.

DIABETES MELLITUS

1. Lungs-fire syndrome ( )

Symptoms:

Dry nose and mouth (4)

Frequent urination (3)

Normal bowel movements (3)

Pain in the throat, also red and swollen (4)

Very thirsty and drink a lot (3)

Vomiting of blood (3)

Treatment principle: to produce fluids and clear heat

Treatment formula: *Xiao-Ke-Fang* and *Jiang-Tang-Yi-Hao-Fang*

Food cures: lily flower, salt, cattail, asparagus, soya milk, duck egg, and olive

2. Stomach-fire syndrome ( )

Symptoms:

Bitter taste in the mouth (1)

Bleeding from gums (1)

Bleeding from space between teeth with pain (1)

Constipation with dry stools (1)

Dry sensations in the mouth (1)

Eating a lot and still feeling hungry (1)

Fever (1)

Headache (1)

Hiccups (1)

Hungry with good appetite and eat a lot, but still underweight (1)

Incapable of sound sleep in children (1)

Morning sickness (1)

Nosebleed (1)

Pain in the gums with swelling (1)

Pain in the throat, also red and swollen (1)

Toothache (1)

Underweight (2)*

Vomiting of blood (1)

Vomiting right after eating (1)

Treatment principle: to sedate fire and nourish the yin and to lubricate dryness

Treatment formula: *Shi-Gao-Zhi-Mu-Jia-Ren-Shen-Tang* and *Jiang-Tang-Er-Hao-Fang*

Food cures: areca nuts, buckwheat, common carp, banana, bitter endive, black fungus, salt, spinach, strawberry, bamboo shoot, cucumber, Job's-tears, liver, leaf beet, mung bean, peppermint, purslane, lily flower, salt, and cattail

3. Kidneys yin deficiency syndrome ( )

Symptoms:

Cough with sputum containing blood or coughing out fresh blood (1)

Dry sensations in the mouth particularly at night (1)

Dry throat (1)

Fatigue (1)

Frequent urination (2)*

Hot sensations in any part of the body (1)

Night sweats (1)

Pain in the heels (1)

Pain in the loins (lumbago) (2)*

Retention of urine (1)

Ringing in ears (1)

Seminal emission with dreams (1)

Sleeplessness (1)

Spots in front of the eyes (1)

Thirst (1)

Toothache or shaky teeth (1)

Urine as thick as fat (2)*

Treatment principle: to strengthen the semen and the kidney yin

Treatment formula: *Liu-Wei-Di-Huang-Wan, Wu-Wei-Di-Huang-Wan,* or *Jiang-Tang-San-Hao-Fang*

Food cures: abalone, asparagus, chicken egg, cuttlefish, duck, duck egg, white fungus, oyster, pork, royal jelly, chestnut, chicken liver, and pork kidneys

CORONARY HEART DISEASE

1. Heart-blood coagulations syndrome ( )

Symptoms:
Chest congestion (5)*
Chronic backache (1)
Cold hands and feet (1)
Excessive perspiration (1)
Pain in the chest (1)
Pain in the heart and chest as if being pricked with a needle (6)*
Pale complexion (1)
Palpitations (1)
Perspire a lot (1)
Poor appetite (1)
Shortness of breath (1)
Treatment principle: to warm the heart yang and promote blood circulation
Treatment formula: Gua-Lou-Xie-Bai-Gui-Zhi-Tang
Food cures: ambergris, brown sugar, chestnut, eggplant, peach, black soybean, sturgeon, sweet basil, crab, distillers' grains, papaya, and saffron

2. Simultaneous energy congestion and blood coagulations syndrome ( )

Symptoms:
Abdominal swelling (1)
Chest pain affecting the back (5)*
Chest pain that comes and goes as if being pricked by a needle (7)*
Congested chest (2)
Liver disease (1)
Love of sighing (1)
Lump in the abdomen that stays in the same region (1)
Shortness of breath (1)
Ulcers (1)
Treatment principle: to activate the blood and promote energy circulation
Treatment formula: Xue-Fu-Zhu-Yu-Tang
Food cures: beef, cherry, bird's nest, butterfish, chicken, coconut meat, date, tofu, mustard seed, sweet rice, goose meat, mutton, jackfruit, squash, sweet potato, red and black date, rice, rock sugar, caraway seed, spearmint, common button mushroom, oregano, red bean, ambergris, dill seed, garlic, sweet basil, saffron, brown sugar, chestnut, eggplant, peach, black soybean, sturgeon, sweet basil, crab, distillers' grains, papaya, and saffron

3. Liver-kidneys yin deficiency syndrome ( )

Symptoms:
Chest pain particularly at night (3)*
Difficulty with both defecation and urination (1)
Dizziness (1)
Dry eyes, throat, or mouth (3)*
Fatigue (1)
Headache with pain in the brow (1)
Lumbago (1)
Menstrual pain (1)
Night blindness (1)
Night sweats (1)
Pain in the upper abdomen (1)
Palms of hands and soles of feet are both hot (1)
Paralysis (1)
Sleeplessness with forgetfulness (1)
Weak loins and tibia (1)

Withering complexion (1)

Treatment principle: to strengthen the kidneys and liver yin and to activate the blood and transform blood coagulations

Treatment formula: *Yang-Yin-Tong-Bi-Tang*

Food cures: bird's nest, cheese, chicken egg, kidney bean, brown sugar, mussel, abalone, asparagus, chicken egg, cuttlefish, duck, duck egg, white fungus, oyster, pork, royal jelly, chestnut, chicken liver, and pork kidneys

4. Simultaneous deficiency of yin and yang syndrome ( )

Symptoms:

Cold limbs and cold sensations in the body (1)

Fatigue (1)

Frequent urination at night (4)*

Low energy (1)

Pain in the heart (3)*

Palpitations (1)

Perspiration with hot sensations in the body easily triggered by physical activities (1)

Poor appetite (1)

Poor spirits (1)

Ringing in ears (1)

Too tired to talk (1)

Underweight (1)

Wake up at night due to pain (3)*

Treatment principle: to regulate and strengthen both the yin and yang and to strengthen the energy and the blood simultaneously

Treatment formula: *Zhi-Gan-Cao-Tang*

Food cures: beef, cherry, bird's nest, butterfish, chicken, coconut meat, date, tofu, mustard seed, sweet rice, goose meat, mutton, jackfruit,

squash, sweet potato, red and black date, rice, rock sugar, caraway seed, spearmint, common button mushroom, oregano, red bean, ambergris, dill seed, garlic, sweet basil, saffron, abalone, asparagus, cuttlefish, chicken egg, duck egg, white fungus, beef liver, grape, mandarin fish, oyster, milk, beef, blood clam, and longan nuts

URINARY STONES

Urinary stones usually display pain across the loins, abdominal pain, prickling pain on urination, and blood in urine

1. Lower burning space dampness-heat syndrome ( )

Symptoms:

Pain affecting the lower abdomen or shooting pain towards the genitals (3)*

Colic pain in the abdomen and across the loins (3)*

Dribbling after urination (3)*

Frequent desire to pass urine (2)*

Frequent urination in short reddish streams (1)

Low fever in the afternoon (1)

Nausea or vomiting (1)

Pain on urination (2)*

Poor appetite (1)

Seminal emission (1)

Thirst with no desire for drink (1)

Yellowish and turbid urine (2)*

Treatment principle: to clear the heat and remove dampness and to expel stones

Treatment formula: *Dao-Chi-San*

Food cures: mung bean sprouts, ambergris, kiwi fruits, sturgeon, adzuki bean, Chinese cabbage, mango, pea, and watermelon

2. Simultaneous energy congestion and blood coagulations syndrome (   )

Symptoms:
Abdominal swelling (1)
Aching pain in the lower abdomen (2)*
Chronic stones (3)*
Colic pain on urination (2)*
Congested chest (1)
Dribbling after urination (3)*
Love of sighing (1)
Lump in the abdomen that stays in the same region (1)
Pain across the loins (3)*
Pain on urination (3)*
Treatment principle: to regulate energy and remove blood coagulations
Treatment formula: *Tao-Hong-Si-Wu-Tang*
Food cures: beef, cherry, bird's nest, butterfish, chicken, coconut meat, date, tofu, mustard seed, sweet rice, goose meat, mutton, jackfruit, squash, sweet potato, red and black date, rice, rock sugar, caraway seed, spearmint, common button mushroom, oregano, red bean, ambergris, dill seed, garlic, sweet basil, saffron, brown sugar, chestnut, eggplant, peach, black soybean, sturgeon, crab, distillers' grains, papaya, and saffron

3. Spleen-kidneys yang deficiency syndrome (   )

Symptoms:
Chronic stones (6)*
Cold hands and feet (1)
Cold loins (1)

Diarrhea before dawn (2)
Diarrhea with sticky, muddy stools (1)
Eating very little (1)
Edema that occurs all over the body (1)
Fatigue (2)
Fear of cold (1)
Four limbs weakness (1)
Frequent urination with clear or white urine (1)
Mentally fatigued (1)
Sputum rumbling with panting (1)
Treatment principle: to strengthen the spleen and the kidneys and to promote urination and expel stones
Treatment formula: *Shen-Ling-Bai-Zhu-San*
Food cures: air bladder of shark, chicken, cayenne pepper, fennel, nutmeg, black and white pepper, prickly ash, mutton, sword bean, white or yellow mustard, kidney, lobster, sardine, shrimp, sparrow, clove, dill seed, fennel, pistachio nut, sparrow egg, crab apple, raspberry, and walnut

ANEMIA

1. Heart-spleen deficiency syndrome (   )

Symptoms:
Abdominal swelling (1)
Bleeding symptoms (2)*
Discharge of watery, thin stools (1)
Dizziness (1)
Eating very little (1)
Fatigue (1)
Fatigue with a lack of power (1)
Forgetfulness (1)
Impotence (1)
Low voice (1)
Nervousness (2)

Night sweats (1)
Palpitations (2)
Poor appetite (1)
Shortness of breath (1)
Sleeplessness (2)
Withering and yellowish complexion (1)

Treatment principle: to strengthen the spleen and the heart and to tone the blood and the energy

Treatment formula: *Gui-Pi-Tang*

Food cures: beef liver, chicken egg, cuttlefish, oyster, pork liver, sea cucumber, water spinach, longan nut, mandarin fish, apple cucumber, chestnut, horse bean, Job's-tears, Irish potato, rice, royal jelly, and yam

2. Liver-kidneys yin deficiency syndrome (   )

Symptoms:
Difficulty in both defecation and urination (1)
Dizziness (2)
Dry eyes or throat (1)
Fatigue (2)
Headache with pain in the brow (1)
Lumbago (2)
Night blindness (1)
Night sweats (1)
Pain in the upper abdomen (2)
Palms of hands and soles of feet are both hot (1)
Red eyes (1)
Ringing in the ears (1)
Sleeplessness with forgetfulness (1)
Weak loins and tibia (1)
Withering complexion (1)
Zygomatic regions on both sides appear tender and red (1)

Treatment principle: to water the liver yin and the kidney yin and to nourish the blood and strengthen the essence of the kidneys

Treatment formula: *Gui-Shao-Di-Huang-Tang*

Food cures: bird's nest, cheese, chicken egg, kidney bean, brown sugar, mussel, abalone, asparagus, chicken egg, cuttlefish, duck, duck egg, white fungus, oyster, pork, royal jelly, chestnut, chicken liver, and pork kidneys

3. Spleen-kidneys yang deficiency syndrome (   )

Symptoms:
Cold hands and feet (2)
Cold loins (2)
Diarrhea before dawn (2)
Diarrhea with sticky and muddy stools (1)
Eating very little (1)
Edema (2)
Edema that occurs all over the body (1)
Fatigue (2)
Fear of cold (1)
Four limbs weakness (1)
Frequent urination with clear or white urine (1)
Mentally fatigued (1)
Pale complexion (1)
Palpitations (1)
Poor appetite (1)
Puffy face (1)
Sputum rumbling with panting (1)

Treatment principle: to strengthen the spleen and the kidneys and to tone the energy and the blood

Treatment formula: *Ren-Shen-Yang-Ying-Tang*

Food cures: air bladder of shark, chicken, cayenne pepper, fennel, nutmeg, black and white pepper, prickly ash, mutton, sword bean, white or yellow mustard, kidney, lobster, sardine, shrimp, sparrow, clove, dill seed, fennel, pistachio nut, sparrow egg, crab apple, raspberry, and walnut

EPILEPSY

1. Wind-sputum syndrome ( )

Symptoms:
Convulsions (1)
Discharge of clear sputum with lots of bubbles (1)
Dizziness (1)
Numbness of the four limbs (1)
Seizures that occur very frequently (2)*
Seizures with a shrill cry (2)*
Seizures with incontinence of both urination and bowel movements (2)*
Seizures with lockjaw or both eyes looking straight up (2)*
Seizures preceded by headache, dizziness, and congested chest (2)*
Sputum noise in the throat (1)
Stiffness of the tongue and unable to talk (1)
Sudden fainting (1)
Tics (1)
Vomiting of clear or white, watery sputum (1)
Wry mouth and eyes (1)
Treatment principle: to expel sputum and relieve seizures
Treatment formula: *Ding-Xian-Wan* or *Xie-Gan-An-Shen-Wan*
Food cures: peppermint, spearmint, sweet basil, celery, coconut meat, green onion, asparagus, bamboo shoot, date, leaf or brown mustard, mustard seed, black and white pepper, fresh ginger, and crown daisy

2. Sputum-fire syndrome ( )

Symptoms:
Bitter taste in the mouth (2)
Constipation (2)
Hungry with no appetite (1)
Insanity (1)
Insomnia (2)
Jumpiness (2)
Presence of sputum difficult to spit out (4)*
Ringing in ears and deafness (1)
Seizures with a shrill cry (2)
Seizures with fainting, convulsions, and vomiting of sputum (3)*
Treatment principle: to clear the heat in the liver and sedate fire and to transform sputum and open the cavities
Treatment formula: *Long-Dan-Xie-Gan-Tang* with *Tiao-Tan-Tang*
Food cures: salt, cattail, agar, radish, bamboo shoot, crown daisy, date, fresh ginger, leaf or brown mustard, black and white pepper, white or yellow mustard seed, asparagus, and pear

3. Heart-kidneys yang deficiency syndrome ( )

Symptoms:
Discharge of watery, thin stools (1)
Edema (1)
Epilepsy with a long history (4)*
Forgetfulness (3)*
Frequent urination (1)
Pain in the chest (2)
Palpitations (2)
Poor appetite (1)
Nervousness (2)
Shock (1)
Speech not clear (1)
Sputum (1)
Treatment principle: to tone the heart and the kidneys and to strengthen the spleen and transform sputum
Treatment formula: *He-Che-Wan* or *Da-Bu-Yuan-Jian* with *Liu-Jun-Zi-Tang*

118

Food cures: dried ginger, cinnamon, wheat, water spinach, kidneys, star anise, red and black date, lobster, sardine, shrimp, sparrow, clove, dill seed, fennel, pistachio nut, sparrow egg, crab apple, raspberry, and walnut

HYPERTHYROIDISM

1. Hot stomach syndrome (   )

Symptoms:
Bad breath (2)
Bleeding from gums (1)
Foul breath from the mouth (1)
Getting hungry easily (1)
Gums swelling (1)
Hiccups (1)
Nosebleed (1)
Pain in the gums with swelling (2)
Pain in the throat (1)
Perspiring on the head (1)
Stomachache (2)
Thirst and craving for cold drink (1)
Underweight (1)
Vomiting (2)
Vomiting of blood (2)
Vomiting right after eating (1)
Treatment principle: to clear the heat in the stomach and disperse the energy in the liver
Treatment formula: *Dao-Chi-Cheng-Qi-Tang*
Food cures: salt, lily flower, bitter endive, camellia, cattail, black fungus, spinach, strawberry, banana, cucumber, and licorice

2. Liver energy congestion syndrome (   )

Symptoms:
Abdominal obstruction (2)
Abdominal pain (2)
Convulsions (1)
Insomnia (2)*

Numbness (1)
Pain in the upper abdomen (2)
Psychological tension (2)*
Stomachache (2)
Subjective sensations of objects in the throat (2)*
Swollen tonsils (2)*
Vomiting of blood (1)
Worry a lot (1)
Treatment principle: to regulate the energy of the liver and to remove sputum and relieve congestion
Treatment formula: *Si-Hai-Shu-Yu-Wan*
Food cures: brown sugar, garlic, turmeric, kumquat, beef, cherry, bird's nest, butterfish, chicken, coconut meat, date, tofu, mustard seed, sweet rice, goose meat, mutton, jackfruit, squash, sweet potato, red and black date, rice, rock sugar, caraway seed, spearmint, common button mushroom, oregano, red bean, ambergris, dill seed, sweet basil, and saffron

3. Sputum-fire syndrome (   )

Symptoms:
Dislike of heat (3)*
Eat a lot (2)*
Emotionally disturbed easily (3)*
Excessive perspiration (2)*
Hungry with no appetite (1)
Insanity (1)
Palpitations (3)*
Ringing in ears and deafness (1)
Sleeplessness (1)
Swollen tonsils (3)*
Treatment principle: to sedate sputum-fire and to nourish the heart and secure the spirits
Treatment formula: *Er-Yin-Jian* with *Ding-Zhi-Wan*
Food cures: salt, cattail, agar, radish, bamboo shoot, crown daisy, date,

fresh ginger, leaf or brown
mustard, black and white pepper,
white or yellow mustard seed,
asparagus, and pear

4. Liver-kidneys yin deficiency syndrome ( )

Symptoms:
Difficulty in both defecation and
urination (1)
Dizziness (3)
Dry eyes or dry throat (1)
Fatigue (3)
Headache with pain in brow (1)
Lumbago (3)
Night blindness (1)
Night sweats (1)
Pain in the upper abdomen (3)
Palms of hands and soles of feet are
both hot (1)
Sleeplessness with forgetfulness (1)
Withering complexion (1)
Treatment principle: to tone the
energy and the yin and to water
the kidneys and nourish the liver
Treatment formula: *Sheng-Mai-San*
with *Yi-Guan-Jian*
Food cures: bird's nest, cheese,
chicken egg, kidney bean, brown
sugar, mussel, abalone, asparagus,
chicken egg, cuttlefish, duck, duck
egg, white fungus, oyster, pork,
royal jelly, chestnut, chicken liver,
and pork kidneys

5. Deficiency fire syndrome ( )

Symptoms:
Becoming angry easily (2)*
Coughing out blood (1)
Dry cough without sputum or
coughing out slightly sticky fluids
(1)
Dry sensations in the mouth (1)

Dry or sore throat (1)
Excessive perspiration (2)*
Feeling miserable (1)
Forgetfulness (1)
Hot sensations in body, including
hands and feet (2)*
Light but periodic fever not unlike
the tide (1)
Night sweats (1)
Red complexion (2)*
Ringing in ears (1)
Seminal emission with dreams (1)
Sleeplessness (1)
Sputum with blood (1)
Treatment principle: to water the
yin, increase body fluids, and clear
the stomach and nourish the lungs
Treatment formula: *Yu-Nü-Jian* with
Zeng-Yi-Tang
Food cures: banana, bitter endive,
black fungus, salt, spinach,
strawberry, bamboo shoot,
cucumber, Job's-tears, liver, leaf
beet, mung bean, peppermint,
purslane, lily flower, salt, cattail,
chicken egg, duck egg, asparagus,
royal jelly, pork, and oyster

6. Simultaneous deficiency of yin and energy syndrome ( )

Symptoms:
Constipation (1)
Dry cough with scant sputum or dry
mouth (1)
Discharge of dry stools (1)
Excessive perspiration (1)
Fatigue (3)*
Hot sensations in the palms of hands
and soles of feet (1)
Light stomachache with swelling (2)
Palpitations (2)
Poor appetite (1)
Ringing in ears (1)
Scant urine (1)

Sore throat (1)
Thirst (3)*
"Tidal" fever in the afternoon (1)
Treatment principle: to strengthen the energy and nourish the yin and to tone the lungs and water the kidneys
Treatment formula: *Di-Huang-Yin-Zi*
Food cures: bird's nest, cheese, kidney bean, abalone, asparagus, chicken egg, cuttlefish, duck, duck egg, white fungus, oyster, pork, royal jelly, grape, longan nuts, maltose, mandarin fish, Irish potato, sweet rice, apple cucumber, bog bean, gold carp, carrot, chestnut, ham, horse bean, hyacinth bean, Job's-tears, royal jelly, string bean, whitefish, yam, red and black date, mutton, squash, and rock sugar

HYPOTHYROIDISM

1. Spleen-kidneys yang deficiency syndrome ( )

Symptoms:
Being physically weak and too tired to talk (1)
Cold hands and feet (1)
Cold loins (1)
Diarrhea before dawn (2)
Diarrhea with sticky and muddy stools (1)
Dysentery (?)
Eating very little (1)
Edema (2)
Edema that occurs all over the body (1)
Fatigue (2)
Fear of cold (1)
Four limbs weakness (1)
Frequent urination with clear or white urine (1)
Impotence in men and irregular menstruation in women (4)*

Mentally fatigued (1)
Sputum rumbling with panting (1)
Treatment principle: to warm the kidneys and strengthen the spleen
Treatment formula: *You-Gui-Wan*
Food cures: air bladder of shark, chicken, cayenne pepper, fennel, nutmeg, black and white pepper, prickly ash, mutton, sword bean, white or yellow mustard, kidneys, lobster, sardine, shrimp, sparrow, clove, dill seed, pistachio nut, sparrow egg, crab apple, raspberry, and walnut

2. Heart-kidneys yang deficiency syndrome ( )

Symptoms:
Chest pain (2)*
Cold limbs (2)*
Discharge of watery, thin stools (1)
Edema (2)
Frequent urination (1)
History of hydropericardium and cardiac insufficiency (2)*
Love of lying down (2)*
Pain in the chest (2)
Palpitations (2)
Nervousness (2)
Shock (1)
Sputum (1)
Treatment principle: to warm the heart yang and strengthen the kidneys energy
Treatment formula: *Ling-Gui-Zhu-Gan-Tang* with *Shen-Qi-Wan*
Food cures: dried ginger, cinnamon, wheat, water spinach, kidneys, star anise, red and black date, lobster, sardine, shrimp, sparrow, clove, dill seed, fennel, pistachio nut, sparrow egg, crab apple, raspberry, and walnut

3. Spleen-kidneys yang deficiency syndrome ( )

Symptoms:
Being physically weak and too tired to talk (1)
Cold hands and feet (1)
Cold loins (1)
Diarrhea before dawn (2)
Diarrhea with sticky and muddy stools (1)
Dysentery (1)
Eating very little (1)
Edema that occurs all over the body (1)
Fatigue (1)
Fear of cold (1)
Feeble breath (2)*
Frequent urination with clear or white urine (1)
History of myxedema (2)*
Low body temperature (2)*
Mentally fatigued (1)
Sputum rumbling with panting (1)
Treatment principle: to strengthen the yang energy and to warm the kidneys and the spleen
Treatment formula: *Si-Ni-Jia-Ren-Shen-Tang*
Food cures: air bladder of shark, chicken, cayenne pepper, fennel, nutmeg, black and white pepper, prickly ash, mutton, sword bean, white or yellow mustard, kidneys, lobster, sardine, shrimp, sparrow, clove, dill seed, pistachio nut, sparrow egg, crab apple, raspberry, and walnuts

4. Simultaneous deficiency of kidneys yin and kidneys yang ( )

Symptoms:
Cough (1)
Decreased sexual desire in men (1)
Dry mouth (2)*
Edema (1)
Fatigue (2)
Grey hair and falling out of hair (1)
Impotence in men (1)
Infertility in women (1)
Lumbago (1)
Mental fatigue (1)
Panting (2)
Thirst (2)
Weakened legs (1)
Yellowish urine (3)*
Treatment principle: to tone both the yin and the yang
Treatment formula: *Zuo-Gui-Wan*
Food cures: abalone, asparagus, chicken egg, cuttlefish, duck, duck egg, white fungus, oyster, pork, royal jelly, chestnut, chicken liver, pork kidneys, lobster, sardine, shrimp, sparrow, clove, dill seed, fennel, pistachio nut, sparrow egg, crab apple, raspberry, and walnut

ARTHRITIS AND RHEUMATOID ARTHRITIS

Arthritis

1. Wind-predominating type ( )

Symptoms:
Diarrhea containing undigested food (1)
Discharge of watery, thin stools (1)
Dislike of wind (1)
Headache accompanied by fear of wind (1)
Headache with heavy sensations in the head (1)
Itchy skin that becomes almost intolerable (1)
Light cough (1)
Nasal discharge (1)
Numbness in the skin of the face (1)
Pain in all the joints that attacks suddenly (3)*

Pain in the joints that shifts from one joint to another (3)*
Shaking of four limbs and body (1)
Sneezing (1)
Stiffness of muscles (1)
Stuffed nose with heavy voice (1)
Tickle in the throat (1)
Treatment principle: to expel the wind, disperse cold, and remove dampness
Treatment formula: *Fang-Feng-Tang*
Food cures: peppermint, spearmint, sweet basil, celery, coconut meat, and green onion

2. Cold-predominating type ( )

Symptoms:
Abdominal pain (1)
Absence of perspiration in hot weather (1)
Absence of thirst in mouth (1)
Abundant watering of eyes (1)
Clear and long streams of urine in large amounts (1)
Cold chest or cold hands and feet (1)
Cold sensations in the body (1)
Contraction of tendons and muscles (1)
Coughing out and vomiting bubbles of water (1)
Diarrhea with sticky and muddy stools (1)
Dislike of cold (1)
Hands and feet extremely cold (1)
Headache with pain in back of neck (1)
Love of hot drink (1)
Pale complexion (1)
Severe pain in the joints (5)*
Treatment principle: to warm the body and disperse cold and to remove wind and dampness
Treatment formula: *Wu-Tou-Tang*

Food cures: cayenne pepper, dill seed, fennel, fresh ginger, mustard seed, prickly ash, star anise, white or yellow mustard, and wine

3. Dampness-predominating type ( )

Symptoms:
Abdominal pain with abdominal rumbling (1)
Diarrhea (1)
Diminished urination (1)
Discharge of hard stool followed by sticky, turbid stool (1)
Discharge of watery pus through openings of carbuncles (1)
Discharge of yellow, sticky fluids from blisters that break open (1)
Dizziness (1)
Eczema (1)
Edema on the dorsum of foot (1)
Four limbs weakness (1)
Headache as if the head were being wrapped up (1)
Heavy sensation in body or in any part of the body (1)
Love of hot drink (1)
Love of sleep and heavy sensations in the body (1)
Pain always in same joints with heavy sensations of the body (2)*
Pain in the loins as if sitting in water with heaviness in body (2)*
Pain starts mostly from lower regions of the body (2)*
Treatment principle: to strengthen the spleen and remove dampness and to expel wind and disperse cold
Treatment formula: *Yi-Yi-Ren-Tang*
Food cures: carp, celery, horse bean, jellyfish skin, Job's-tears, prickly ash, hyacinth bean, oregano, sweet basil, adzuki bean, bamboo shoot, soybean sprouts, and rosin

4. Heat-predominating type ( )

Symptoms:
Acute onset of pain in the joints (1)
Constipation (1)
Diminished urination (1)
Discharge of copious, yellow, sticky sputum (1)
Dry lips or teeth (1)
Escape of gas from the anus with noise (1)
Light fever (1)
Love of cold drink (1)
Pain in the joints that shifts around (2)*
Pain in the joints with burning sensations (2)*
Pain very severe with inability to extend or flex the joints (2)*
Red complexion, red eyes, or red urine (1)
Short streams of scant urine (1)
Stools with an extremely bad smell (1)
Thirst with an incessant desire to drink (1)
Throat swollen and red, producing rotten liquid (1)
Urine with an extremely bad smell (1)
Treatment principle: to clear heat and to expel wind and remove dampness
Treatment formula: *Bai-Hu-Jia-Gui-Zhi-Tang*
Food cures: banana, bitter endive, black fungus, salt, spinach, strawberry, bamboo shoot, cucumber, Job's-tears, laver, leaf beet, mung bean, peppermint, and purslane

Rheumatoid Arthritis

1. Wind-cold-dampness type ( )

Symptoms:
Joints neither red nor burning (5)*
Pain affected by change in weather (5)*
Pain gets worse when cold and better when warm (2)
Pain involving one or two joints only (5)*
Arthritis with a shorter history (2)
Stiffness of joints more severe in the morning (1)
Treatment principle: to warm the body and disperse cold and to expel dampness and disperse wind
Treatment formula: *Juan-Bi-Tang*
Food cures: peppermint, (including oil), spearmint, sweet basil, cayenne pepper, fennel, fresh ginger, mustard seed, star anise, and prickly ash leaf

2. Heat-excess yin-deficiency type ( )

Symptoms:
Bitter taste in the mouth (3)
Dry mouth (3)
Joints swollen and painful with burning sensations (3)
Arthritis with a longer history (5)*
Pain gets better with coolness at the beginning, then gradually gets better with warmth (3)
Stiffness of joints (3)
Treatment principle: to disperse cold and remove dampness and to transform sputum and activate the blood
Treatment formula: *Gui-Zhi-Shao-Yao-Zhi-Mu-Tang*

Food cures: banana, bitter endive, black fungus, salt, spinach, strawberry, bamboo shoot, cucumber, Job's-tears, laver, leaf beet, mung bean, peppermint, and purslane

3. Deficiency type (   )

Symptoms:
Breathing with a low sound and feeble breath (1)
Chronic pain in the joints over a long duration (2)*
Eating very little (1)
Feeble voice with intermittent speech (1)
Hiccups that are slow and occur infrequently (1)
Hoarseness (1)
Light and clear voice with low and feeble tone (1)
Little power (1)
Pain in inner part of stomach that lessens after meals, and desire for massage (1)
Pain in the joints that is more severe at night (3)*
Prolonged dizziness (1)
Retention of urine (1)
Scant and handicapped breathing (1)
Scant breathing that becomes intermittent when talking too much (1)
Small breaths (1)
Talking in weak voice (1)
Underweight (1)
Treatment principle: to strengthen the kidneys and the body energy and to promote energy and blood circulation to relieve pain
Treatment formula: *Juan-Bi-Tang*
Food cures: soya milk, goose meat, milk, royal jelly, grape, longan nuts, mandarin fish, milk, maltose, and Irish potato

COMMON COLD AND FLU

1. Wind-cold syndrome (   )

Symptoms:
Absence of perspiration in hot weather (1)
Breathing through the nose (1)
Clear discharge from nose (1)
Cough with heavy, unclear sounds and clear sputum (1)
Diarrhea (1)
Dislike of cold (3)*
Dizziness (1)
Headache with dizziness (1)
Hoarseness at the beginning of illness (1)
Itch in the throat (1)
Light fever (2)*
Loss of voice (1)
Nosebleed (1)
Pain in the body shifting around with no fixed region (1)
Pain in the joints (1)
Stuffed nose (1)
Vomiting (1)
Treatment principle: to induce perspiration and expand the lungs and to disperse cold
Treatment formula: *Jing-Fang-Bai-Du-San*
Food cures: peppermint (including oil), spearmint, sweet basil, cayenne pepper, fennel, fresh ginger, mustard seed, star anise, and prickly ash leaf

2. Wind-heat syndrome (   )

Symptoms:
Coughing out yellowish sputum (2)*
Fever appears more severe than chills (2)*
Headache with dizziness (1)
Intolerance of light in eyes with swelling and dislike of wind (1)
Muddy discharge from nose (1)

Nosebleed (1)
Pain in the eyes (1)
Pain in the throat (2)*
Perspiration (4)*
Red eyes (1)
Thirst (1)
Toothache (1)
Yellow urine (1)
Yellowish discharge from the nose (1)
Treatment principle: to induce perspiration and clear heat
Treatment formula: *Yin-Qiao-San*
Food cures: banana, bitter endive, black fungus, salt, spinach, strawberry, bamboo shoot, cucumber, Job's-tears, laver, leaf beet, mung bean, peppermint, purslane, spearmint, sweet basil, celery, coconut meat, and green onion

3. Summer heat syndrome ( )

Symptoms:
Chest discomfort (1)
Constipation (1)
Cough (1)
Dizziness (2)*
Dry lips or dry sensations in the mouth (1)
Fatigue (1)
Feeling miserable and thirsty (1)
Heavy sensations in the head (1)
High fever (2)*
Nausea and vomiting (1)
No perspiration (2)*
Obstructed urination with red urine (1)
Oppressed and rapid breath (1)
Perspiration due to hot weather or putting on warm clothes (1)
Perspire a lot (1)
Scant and reddish urine (1)
Thirst (1)
Treatment principle: to clear summer heat and transform dampness with aromatic herbs

Treatment formula: *Xin-Jia-Xiang-Ru-Yin*
Food cures: apple, apple cucumber, cantaloupe, coconut liquid, hyacinth bean, lemon, watermelon, banana, bamboo shoot, bitter endive, bitter gourd, celery, chicken egg white, crab, mung bean, peppermint, and purslane

BACILLARY DYSENTERY

Acute Bacillary Dysentery

1. Superficial dampness-heat syndrome ( )

Symptoms:
Abdominal pain (2)*
Congested chest (2)*
Diarrhea with forceful discharge of stools (1)
Discharge of yellowish-red, turbid stools with bad smell (1)
Excessive perspiration (1)
Greasy taste in the mouth (2)*
Jaundice (2)
Low fever (1)
Pain in the joints of the four limbs, with swelling and heaviness (1)
Perspiration on hands and feet or the head (1)
Reddish and scant urine (1)
Retention of urine (1)
Swollen body of the tongue (1)
Thirst with no desire for drink (2)*
Yellowish body (1)
Treatment principle: to clear heat and remove dampness and to regulate energy and harmonize the blood
Treatment formula: *Shao-Yao-Tang*
Food cures: carp, celery, horse bean, jellyfish skin, Job's-tears, prickly ash, hyacinth bean, oregano, sweet basil, adzuki bean, bamboo

126

shoot, soybean sprouts, rosin, banana, bitter endive, black fungus, salt, spinach, strawberry, cucumber, leaf beet, mung bean, peppermint, and purslane

2. Heat poisoning penetrating into the deep regions syndrome ( )

Symptoms:
Acute abdominal pain (2)*
Acute onset of symptoms (2)*
Breathing difficulty (1)
Cold and hot sensations together (1)
Discharge of pus and blood from anus (2)*
Discharge of blood from the mouth (1)
Headache that is severe (1)
High fever (2)*
Misty vision (1)
Nosebleed (1)
Not alert (1)
Severe pain in whole body (1)
Twitching (1)
Very difficult bowel movements (2)*
Vomiting of blood (1)
Treatment principle: to clear heat and remove dampness and to cool the blood and counteract poisoning
Treatment formula: Ge-Gan-Qin-Lian-Tang
Food cures: adzuki bean, banana, bitter endive, bitter gourd, chicken egg white, chicken gallbladder, cucumber, fig, mung bean, black and white pepper, peppermint, squash, and strawberry

Chronic Bacillary Dysentery

1. Spleen yang deficiency syndrome ( )

Symptoms:
Abdominal pain (3)*

Chronic bowel movement difficulty (3)*
Cold in the forehead that does not warm up (1)
Dysentery with discharge of pus and blood (3)*
Edema (2)
Hot sensations with nausea (3)*
Intermittent diarrhea (3)*
Stomachache (2)
Treatment principle: to warm the spleen yang and to clear heat and remove dampness
Treatment formula: Huang-Lian-Tang
Food cures: air bladder of shark, chicken, cayenne pepper, fennel, nutmeg, black and white pepper, prickly ash, mutton, sword bean, and white or yellow mustard

BRONCHITIS

Acute Bronchitis

1. Cold-wind restricting the lungs syndrome ( )

Symptoms:
Common cold (2)
Cough with heavy, unclear sounds and clear sputum (3)*
Dislike of cold (1)
Fever (3)*
Headache (1)
Itch in the throat (1)
Lack of perspiration (1)
Nasal congestion (3)*
Nasal discharge (3)*
Panting (2)
Treatment principle: to disperse wind and cold and to expand the lungs and stop cough
Treatment formula: Xing-Su-San
Food cures: almond, rock sugar, asparagus, peppermint (including oil), spearmint, sweet basil, cayenne pepper, fennel, fresh

ginger, mustard seed, star anise, prickly ash leaf, leaf or brown mustard, walnut, common button mushroom, and tangerine

2. Wind-heat offending the lungs syndrome (   )

Symptoms:
Common cold (1)
Coughing out yellow and sticky sputum (2)*
Dislike of wind (1)
Fever (3)*
Flickering nostrils (1)
Headache (1)
Pain in the chest (1)
Pain in the throat (1)
Perspiration (3)*
Sore throat (3)*
Sputum with blood (2)
Thirst in the mouth with a desire for drink (1)
Treatment principle: to expel wind and clear heat and to expand the lungs and stop cough
Treatment formula: Sang-Ju-Yin (1)
Food cures: apple, apple cucumber, sweet rice, lemon, sweet potato, tofu, tomato, white sugar, coriander, and parsley

3. Lungs-dryness syndrome (   )

Symptoms:
Coughing out blood (1)
Dry cough (3)*
Dry cough without sputum or coughing out slightly sticky fluids (3)*
Dry nose (1)
Dry throat (1)
Dryness in mouth and nose (1)
Loss of voice (1)
Morbid hunger (2)

Thirst (2)
Nosebleed (2)
Pain in the throat (1)
Presence of sputum that can't be coughed out easily (1)
Tickle in the throat (1)
Treatment principle: to clear heat and produce fluids and to lubricate dryness-lungs and rescue the lungs
Treatment formula: Qing-Re-Jiu-Fei-Tang
Food cures: almond, apple, apricot, asparagus, white fungus, licorice, loquat, peanut, pear peel, rock sugar, and tangerine

Chronic Bronchitis

1. Spleen-dampness offending the lungs syndrome (   )

Symptoms:
Cough (3)
Discharge of sputum that can be coughed out easily (1)
Discharge of white, watery sputum (2)
Fatigue of the four limbs (2)
Heavy sensations in head as if head were wrapped up (2)
Heavy sensations in the limbs and trunk (2)
Inability to lie on back (2)
Poor appetite (2)
Short breath (2)
Swelling of hands and feet (1)
Vomiting (1)
Treatment principle: to strengthen the spleen, dry dampness, transform sputum, and regulate the lungs
Treatment formula: Er-Chen-Tang
Food cures: gold carp, corncob, horse bean, Job's-tears, prickly ash, adzuki bean, bamboo shoot,

cheese, ambergris, barley, common carp, cucumber, mung bean, seaweed, shepherd's purse, and star fruit

2. Liver-fire attacking the lungs syndrome ( )

Symptoms:
Cough that causes pain in the upper abdomen (5)*
Cough with sticky sputum (1)
Coughing out blood (2)
Dry throat (1)
Painful sensations running through chest and ribs (1)
Rapid breath (1)
Red face (2)
Sputum with blood (2)
Thirst (1)
Vomiting of blood (4)
Treatment principle: to calm the liver, sedate fire, and clear the heat in the lungs and stop cough
Treatment formula: Ke-Xue-Fang
Food cures: asparagus, soya milk, duck egg, olive, spinach, chestnut, shepherd's purse, rye, black fungus, vinegar, abalone, asparagus, chicken egg, white fungus, pork, and royal jelly

BRONCHIAL ASTHMA

1. Cold sputum obstructing the lungs syndrome ( )

Symptoms:
Cold limbs (1)
Congested chest with a choking sensation (1)
Cough out thin and watery sputum (5)*
Love of hot or warm drink (1)
No perspiration (1)
Pain in the chest (3)
Panting (3)

Swelling of the lungs (1)
Wheezing (4)*
Treatment principle: to warm the lungs and expel cold and to remove sputum
Treatment formula: She-Gan-Ma-Huang-Tang
Food cures: fresh ginger, leaf or brown mustard, black and white pepper, and white or yellow mustard seed

2. Sputum-heat accumulated in the lungs syndrome ( )

Symptoms:
Acute respiration, and gasping for air (2)
Cough out yellowish or sticky sputum (7)*
Panting (3)
Swelling of the lungs (3)
Thirst with craving for cold drink (1)
Wheezing (4)
Treatment principle: to expand the lungs, clear heat, transform sputum, and push down the lungs energy
Treatment formula: Ma-Xing-Shi-Gan-Tang
Food cures: apple peel, common button mushroom, grapefruit peel, radish, and pear

3. Lungs-dampness syndrome ( )

Symptoms:
Congested chest (2)
Copious, sticky sputum (4)*
Cough with gasping for air (2)
Insomnia (2)
Nausea (2)
Palpitations (2)
Poor appetite (2)
Vomiting (2)

Underweight (2)

Treatment principle: to push down lungs energy, transform sputum, promote energy circulation, and stop panting and cough

Treatment formula: *San-Zi-Tang* with *Er-Chen-Tang*

Food cures: cheese, Job's-tears, adzuki bean, ambergris, barley, bamboo shoot, common carp, cucumber, mung bean, seaweed, shepherd's purse, and star fruit

4. Lungs unable to push down energy syndrome (   )

Symptoms:
Cough (1)
Discharge of copious, whitish, and sticky sputum (3)*
Dislike of cold (1)
Dry throat but without thirst (1)
Inability to lie on back (1)
More exhaling than inhaling (3)*
Pain in the throat (1)
Palpitations (1)
Short streams of reddish urine (1)
Swelling of the lower abdomen (1)
Wheezing that persists or occurs all of a sudden (3)*
Wheezing triggered or intensified by moving around (3)*

Treatment principle: to push down upsurging lungs energy, transform sputum, and relieve panting

Treatment formula: *Shen-Zhe-Zhen-Qi-Tang*

Food cures: adzuki bean, ambergris, barley, bamboo shoot, seaweed, black soybean, almond, areca nut, buckwheat, common carp, cashew nut, coriander, grapefruit peel, loquat, malt, nutmeg, pea, black and white pepper, radish, rice bran, sword bean, and clove

5. Lungs energy deficiency syndrome (   )

Symptoms:
Breathing difficulty (1)
Cold limbs (1)
Common cold (2)
Copious, clear, and watery sputum (1)
Cough (2)
Excessive perspiration (1)
Fatigue (2)
Fear of cold (1)
Dislike of wind (1)
Light wheezing (2)
Low and weak voice (1)
Shortness of breath (1)
Smooth urination (1)
Swelling of the lungs (2)
Too tired to talk (1)

Treatment principle: to strengthen lungs energy, solidify the superficial region, and relieve panting and cough

Treatment formula: *Bu-Fei-Tang*

Food cures: cheese, Job's-tears, yam, grape, longan nut, maltose, mandarin fish, Irish potato, sweet rice, apple cucumber, bog bean, gold carp, carrot, chestnut, ham, horse bean, hyacinth bean, royal jelly, string bean, whitefish, yam, red and black date, mutton, squash, and rock sugar

6. Loss of the kidneys capacity for absorbing inspiration syndrome (   )

Symptoms:
Breathing difficulty (1)
Cold limbs (1)
Fear of cold (1)
Frequent fear of cold both in hands and feet (1)
Frequent urination (3)*

More inhaling than exhaling (2)*
Panting that is triggered or
  intensified by moving around (3)*
Perspiration due to hot weather or
  putting on warm clothes (1)
Shortness of breath (1)
Swelling of the lungs (2)
Wheezing (2)
Whitish sputum (2)*
Treatment principle: to tone and
  warm the kidneys
Treatment formula: *Shen-Qi-Wan*
Food cures: abalone, asparagus,
  chicken egg, cuttlefish, duck, duck
  egg, white fungus, milk, lobster,
  oyster, pork, royal jelly, chestnut,
  chicken liver, pork kidneys,
  sardine, shrimp, sparrow, clove,
  dill seed, fennel, pistachio nut,
  sparrow egg, crab apple,
  raspberry, and walnut

PNEUMONIA

1. Wind-warm-superficial syndrome ( )

Symptoms:
Acute onset of symptoms (4)*
Cough (2)
Dry mouth or thirst (4)*
Fear of cold (1)
High fever (4)*
Light thirst (1)
Nasal discharge (1)
Slight dislike of cold (1)
Stuffy nose (1)
Wheezing from the throat (1)
Treatment principle: to induce
  perspiration with pungent and
  cool herbs, to expand the lungs
  and transform sputum
Treatment formula: *Yin-Qiao-San*
Food cures: apple, apple cucumber,
  sweet rice, lemon, sweet potato,
  tofu, tomato, white sugar,
  coriander, and parsley

2. Sputum energy heat syndrome ( )

Symptoms:
Cough and panting (1)
Coughing out sputum containing
  silky blood (1)
Discharge of copious, yellow, and
  sticky sputum (1)
Dry mouth with desire to wash
  mouth, not to drink (1)
High fever that does not go down for
  a prolonged period of time (2)*
Light cough (1)
Oppressed and rapid breath (1)
Scanty urine (1)
Shivering (3)*
Sputum of a rusty color (2)*
Thirst (2)*
Wheezing with sputum noise (3)*
Treatment principle: to clear heat
  and expand the lungs and to
  transform sputum and push down
  the upsurging energy of the lungs
Treatment formula: *Ma-Xing-Shi-
  Gan-Tang* with *Wei-Jing-Tang*
Food cures: banana, bitter endive,
  black fungus, salt, spinach,
  strawberry, bamboo shoot,
  cucumber, Job's-tears, laver, leaf
  beet, mung bean, peppermint,
  purslane, salt, cattail, agar, radish,
  crown daisy, date, fresh ginger,
  leaf or brown mustard, black and
  white pepper, white or yellow
  mustard seed, asparagus, and pear

3. Heat enters the pericardium syndrome ( )

Symptoms:
Being slow and dull in response (2)
Chest pain (3)*
Difficulty in speech (1)
High fever (3)*
Illusive hearing (1)

Illusive vision (1)
Incontinence of both bowel movements and urination (1)
Indifferent in expression (1)
Mental dizziness (1)
Slightly cold limbs (3)*
Sputum noise in the throat (3)*
Twitching (1)

Treatment principle: to expand the lungs and transform sputum and to clear the heat in the heart and promote blood circulation throughout the whole body

Treatment formula: *Wei-Jing-Tang* with *Qing-Gong-Tang*

Food cures: asparagus, pear peel, banana, bitter endive, black fungus, salt, spinach, strawberry, bamboo shoot, cucumber, Job's-tears, liver, leaf beet, mung bean, peppermint, purslane, lily flower, salt, and cattail

4. Extreme heat generating wind syndrome (   )

Symptoms:
Convulsions (3)*
Fainting (1)
Feeling troubled, quick-tempered, and insecure (1)
High fever (3)*
Muscular tightening (1)
Neck stiffness (1)
Red complexion (3)*
Stiff neck and limbs (3)*
Twitching or spasms of the four limbs (3)*
Wry and shivering tongue (1)

Treatment principle: to nourish the yin and clear heat and to calm the liver and stop the internal wind

Treatment formula: *Ling-Jiao-Gou-Teng-Tang* with *Qing-Ying-Tang*

Food cures: peppermint, spearmint, sweet basil, celery, coconut meat,

green onion, chicken egg, bitter endive, camellia, cattail, black fungus, salt, spinach, strawberry, banana, bamboo shoot, crab, and water clam

ACUTE GASTROENTERITIS

1. Cold-dampness syndrome (   )

Symptoms:
Abdominal pain with rumbling (2)*
Absence of perspiration in hot weather (1)
Acute attack of vomiting and diarrhea (2)*
Clear and watery vaginal discharge with fishy smell (1)
Cold sensations in lower abdomen–genitals region (1)
Cough (1)
Coughing out sputum with a low sound (1)
Diarrhea with discharge of watery stool without offensive smell (3)*
Discharge of sputum that can be coughed out easily (1)
Edema in the four limbs (1)
Headache (1)
Movement difficulty (1)
Pain in the body (1)
Pain in the joints (1)
Scant and clear urine (1)
Stomachache (1)

Treatment principle: to transform dampness-sputum with aromatic herbs and to disperse cold and dry dampness

Treatment formula: *Huo-Xiang-Zheng-Qi-San*

Food cures: cayenne pepper, dill seed, fennel, fresh ginger, mustard seed, prickly ash, star anise, white or yellow mustard, wine, carp, celery, horse bean, jellyfish skin,

Job's-tears, hyacinth bean, oregano, sweet basil, adzuki bean, bamboo shoot, soybean sprouts, and rosin

2. Summer heat and dampness syndrome (   )

Symptoms:
Abdominal fullness (1)
Burning sensation in the anus (2)*
Chest discomfort (1)
Diarrhea (1)
Fever (2)*
Forceful discharge of stools during defecation (3)*
Lack of appetite (1)
Perspiration due to hot weather or putting on warm clothes (1)
Reddish urine (1)
Sudden attack of vomiting and diarrhea (3)*
Thirst (1)
Vomiting of substances with acid (2)*
Yellowish and watery stools (1)

Treatment principle: to clear heat and remove dampness and to regulate the stomach and intestines

Treatment formula: *Ge-Gen-Qin-Lian-Tang*

Food cures: banana, bamboo shoot, bitter endive, bitter gourd, celery, chicken egg white, crab, cucumber, mung bean, peppermint, purslane, carp, horse bean, jellyfish skin, Job's-tears, prickly ash, hyacinth bean, oregano, sweet basil, adzuki bean, soybean sprouts, and rosin

3. Stomach indigestion syndrome (   )

Symptoms:
Abdominal pain or swelling that lessens after bowel movement (3)*

Acid swallowing and belching of bad breath (2)
Belching with poor appetite (3)*
Discharge of watery, thin stools (1)
Insomnia (1)
Sour and bad breath from mouth (1)
Stomachache (2)
Stools with an extremely bad smell (3)*
Vomiting and diarrhea simultaneously (3)*
Vomiting of sour and bad-smelling foods, with a love of cold drink (1)

Treatment principle: to promote digestion and regulate the stomach and intestine

Treatment formula: *Bao-He-Wan*

Food cures: asafoetida, buckwheat, castor bean, jellyfish, malt, peach, radish, water chestnut, cardamon seed, cayenne pepper, coriander, grapefruit, jackfruit, malt, sweet basil, tea, and tomato

4. Spleen-stomach yang deficiency syndrome (   )

Symptoms:
Abdominal pain (2)*
Clear urine (2)*
Cold limbs (1)
Diarrhea and vomiting that occur frequently (2)*
Fatigue (1)
Intermittent hiccups with low sound (1)
Love of warmth and massage (1)
Pain gets worse with fatigue and hunger and better with rest and eating (1)
Pale complexion (1)
Perspiration with cold limbs (2)*
Poor appetite (1)
Shortness of breath (1)
Stomachache (1)

Upset stomach (1)
Vomiting of undigested foods (1)
Water noise in the stomach (1)

Treatment principle: to warm the middle region and disperse cold and to strengthen the spleen and the stomach

Treatment formula: *Fu-Zi-Li-Zhong-Wan*

Food cures: air bladder of shark, chicken, cayenne pepper, fennel, nutmeg, black and white pepper, prickly ash, mutton, sword bean, white or yellow mustard, cardamon seed, carp, cinnamon, garlic, and beef

CHRONIC GASTRITIS AND PEPTIC ULCERS

1. Stomach indigestion syndrome ( )

Symptoms:
Abdominal pain or swelling that lessens after bowel movement (3)*
Acid swallowing and belching of bad breath (1)
Belching with poor appetite (2)*
Discharge of watery, thin stools (1)
Dry stools (2)*
Hot sensations in the body (1)
Insomnia (1)
Red complexion (1)
Sour and bad breath from mouth (1)
Stomachache that worsens on pressure of hand (2)*
Stools with an extremely bad smell (2)*
Vomiting and diarrhea simultaneously (2)*
Vomiting of sour and bad-smelling foods, with a love of cold drink (1)

Treatment principle: to promote digestion and harmonize the stomach

Treatment formula: *Bao-He-Wan*

Food cures: asafoetida, buckwheat, castor bean, jellyfish, malt, peach, radish, water chestnut, cardamon seed, cayenne pepper, coriander, grapefruit, jackfruit, malt, sweet basil, tea, and tomato

2. Liver energy offending the stomach syndrome ( )

Symptoms:
Abdominal rumbling (1)
Belching (3)
Chest discomfort (1)
Hiccups (3)
Irregular bowel movements (1)
Pain in inner part of stomach (2)
Painful sensations running through ribs on both sides (2)
Stomachache that worsens with emotional disturbances (6)*
Vomiting of acid or blood (1)

Treatment principle: to disperse the liver energy and harmonize the stomach

Treatment formula: *Si-Ni-San*

Food cures: carp, celery, corn silk, brown sugar, sweet orange, kumquat, barley, peanut, red and black date, chestnut, and white fungus

3. Stomach yin deficiency syndrome ( )

Symptoms:
Burning pain in stomach (1)
Constipation (1)
Dry cough (1)
Dry lips (1)
Dry sensations in the mouth with craving for drink (2)*
Dysphagia (1)
Hiccups (1)

Hot sensations in the limbs (1)
Indigestion (1)
Insomnia (1)
Light but periodic fever not unlike the tide (1)
Low fever (1)
No appetite (1)
Palpitations (1)
Stomachache that worsens on an empty stomach (2)*
Vomiting (2)*
Vomiting of blood (1)
Treatment principle: to strengthen the stomach and tone the stomach yin energy and to clear the heat in the stomach and push down the upsurging energy of the stomach
Treatment formula: *Mai-Men-Dong-Tang*
Food cures: alfalfa, ginseng leaf, bird's nest, cheese, kidney bean, abalone, asparagus, chicken egg, cuttlefish, duck, duck egg, white fungus, oyster, pork, royal jelly

4. Spleen-stomach yang deficiency syndrome (   )

Symptoms:
Abdominal pain (1)
Cold limbs (2)*
Diarrhea (1)
Fatigue (1)
Intermittent hiccups with low sound (1)
Love of warmth and massage (2)*
Pain worsens with fatigue and hunger (1)
Pain improves with rest and eating (1)
Poor appetite (1)
Shortness of breath (1)
Stomachache with dull pain (2)*
Upset stomach (1)
Vomiting of undigested foods, acid, or clear water (3)*

Water noise in the stomach (1)
Withered and yellowish complexion (1)
Treatment principle: to strengthen the spleen and the stomach and to warm the middle region and expel cold
Treatment formula: *Li-Zhong-Tang*
Food cures: air bladder of shark, chicken, cayenne pepper, fennel, nutmeg, black and white pepper, prickly ash, mutton, sword bean, white or yellow mustard, cardamon seed, carp, cinnamon, garlic, and beef

5. Stomach blood-coagulations syndrome (   )

Symptoms:
Feeling of emptiness and sickness in abdomen (2)
Pain worsens with massage (2)
Pain in inner part of stomach with prickling sensation and swelling (5)*
Pain in inner part of stomach that is acute after meals, with aversion to massage (2)
Pain in fixed region without shifting around (6)*
Vomiting of blood (3)
Treatment principle: to activate the blood and transform blood coagulations and to harmonize the stomach and relieve pain
Treatment formula: *Jia-Wei-Shi-Xiao-San*
Food cures: saffron, ambergris, brown sugar, chestnut, eggplant, peach, black soybean, sturgeon, sweet basil, crab, distillers' grains, and papaya

NEPHRITIS

Acute Nephritis

1. Cold-wind restricting the lungs syndrome ( )

Symptoms:
Common cold (2)
Cough with heavy, unclear sounds and clear sputum (1)
Dislike of cold (3)*
Dry stools (1)
Edema in the head, face, and four limbs (2)*
Fever (2)*
Headache (1)
Itch in the throat (1)
Lack of perspiration (1)
Nasal congestion (1)
Nasal discharge (1)
Panting (2)
Scant and yellowish urine (1)
Thirst (1)
Treatment principle: to expand the lungs, induce perspiration, and promote energy circulation
Treatment formula: *Yue-Bi-Tang*
Food cures: almond, rock sugar, asparagus, peppermint (including oil), spearmint, sweet basil, cayenne pepper, fennel, fresh ginger, mustard seed, star anise, prickly ash leaf, leaf or brown mustard, walnut, common button mushroom, and tangerine

2. Wind-heat offending the lungs syndrome ( )

Symptoms:
Common cold (1)
Cough (1)
Coughing out yellow and sticky sputum (1)
Dry stools (1)
Fever (2)*
Flickering of nostrils (1)
Headache (2)*
Light edema in the four limbs, gradually becoming more severe (2)*
Pain in the chest (1)
Pain in the throat (1)
Scant and reddish urine (2)*
Sputum with blood (2)
Sore throat (2)*
Thirst in the mouth with a desire for drink (1)
Treatment principle: to expand the lungs and clear the heat in the lungs and to promote urination
Treatment formula: *Yin-Qiao-San*
Food cures: apple, apple cucumber, sweet rice, lemon, sweet potato, tofu, tomato, white sugar, coriander, and parsley

3. Dampness heat syndrome ( )

Symptoms:
Dry mouth (2)
Frequent urination in short, reddish streams (2)
Light edema (5)*
Sore throat with pus in the back of the throat (5)*
Swollen tonsils (6)*
Treatment principle: to water and nourish the kidney yin and to clear heat and detoxicate
Treatment formula: *Xiao-Ji-Yin-Zi*
Food cures: mung bean sprouts, ambergris, kiwi fruit, sturgeon, adzuki bean, Chinese cabbage, mango, pea, and watermelon

Chronic Nephritis

1. Spleen-dampness offending the lungs syndrome ( )

Symptoms:
Abdominal swelling with watery stools (1)

Cough (1)

Discharge of sputum that can be coughed out easily (1)

Discharge of white, watery sputum (1)

Fatigue of the four limbs (1)

Fear of cold (2)*

Heavy sensations in head as if head were wrapped up (1)

Heavy sensations in the limbs and trunk (1)

Inability to lie on back (1)

Perspiration or light perspiration (2)*

Poor appetite (1)

Severe edema particularly in the head and face and the upper half of body (3)*

Shortness of breath (1)

Sore throat (1)

Swelling of hands and feet (1)

Vomiting (1)

Treatment principle: to expand the lungs, strengthen the spleen, and reduce edema

Treatment formula: *Yue-Bi-Jia-Zhu-Tang* with *Ma-Huang-Lian-Qiao-Chi-Xiao-Dou-Tang*

Food cures: gold carp, corncob, horse bean, Job's-tears, prickly ash, adzuki bean, bamboo shoot, cheese, ambergris, barley, common carp, cucumber, mung bean, seaweed, shepherd's purse, and star fruit

2. Spleen-kidneys yang deficiency syndrome ( )

Symptoms:

Abdominal swelling like a drum (2)*

Ascites (1)

Being physically weak and too tired to talk (1)

Cold hands and feet (1)

Cold loins (1)

Diarrhea before dawn (2)

Diarrhea with sticky and muddy stools (1)

Edema that occurs all over the body (2)*

Fatigue (2)

Fear of cold (1)

Four limbs weakness (1)

Frequent urination in clear or white streams (1)

Mentally fatigued (1)

Poor appetite (1)

Scant and clear urine (1)

Sputum rumbling with panting (1)

Treatment principle: to warm the spleen and kidneys yang and to promote energy circulation and urination

Treatment formula: *Shi-Pi-Yin*

Food cures: air bladder of shark, chicken, cayenne pepper, fennel, nutmeg, black and white pepper, prickly ash, mutton, sword bean, white or yellow mustard, kidneys, lobster, sardine, shrimp, sparrow, clove, dill seed, pistachio nut, sparrow egg, crab apple, raspberry, and walnut

3. Simultaneous deficiency of energy and blood syndrome ( )

Symptoms:

Abdominal swelling followed by severe edema (3)*

Bleeding of various kinds with blood in light color, often seen in consumptive diseases (1)

Dizziness (1)

Edema that appears only slightly depressed on finger pressure (2)*

Fatigue (2)

Flying objects seen in front of the eyes (1)

Insomnia (2)

Low energy (1)

Low voice (1)
Numbness of limbs (2)*
Pale complexion and lips (1)
Pale nails (1)
Palpitations (1)
Scant urine (1)
Treatment principle: to tone energy and blood simultaneously
Treatment formula: *Shi-Quan-Da-Bu-Wan*
Food cures: abalone, asparagus, cuttlefish, chicken egg, duck egg, white fungus, beef liver, grape, mandarin fish, oyster, milk, beef, cherry, blood clam, longan nut, maltose, Irish potato, sweet rice, apple cucumber, bog bean, gold carp, carrot, chestnut, ham, horse bean, hyacinth bean, Job's-tears, royal jelly, string bean, whitefish, yam, red and black date, mutton, squash, and rock sugar

4. Spleen-kidneys yang deficiency syndrome (   )

Symptoms:
Ascites (1)
Being physically weak and too tired to talk (1)
Cold hands and feet (1)
Cold loins (1)
Diarrhea before dawn (1)
Diarrhea with sticky and muddy stools (1)
Dysentery (2)
Eating very little (1)
Edema (1)
Edema that occurs all over the body (1)
Fatigue (1)
Fear of cold (1)
Four limbs weakness (1)
Frequent urination in clear or white streams (1)
Mentally fatigued (1)

Proteins in the urine (3)*
Sputum rumbling with panting (1)
Treatment principle: to strengthen the spleen and the kidneys yang
Treatment formula: *Shen-Qi-Wan* with *Wu-Zi-Yan-Zong-Wan*
Food cures: air bladder of shark, chicken, cayenne pepper, fennel, nutmeg, black and white pepper, prickly ash, mutton, sword bean, white or yellow mustard, kidneys, lobster, sardine, shrimp, sparrow, clove, dill seed, pistachio nut, sparrow egg, crab apple, raspberry, and walnuts

5. Liver-kidneys yin deficiency syndrome (   )

Symptoms:
Blurred vision (2)*
Difficulty in both defecation and urination (1)
Dizziness (1)
Dry eyes (1)
Dry throat (1)
Fatigue (1)
Headache with pain in the brow (2)*
Lumbago (1)
Night blindness (1)
Night sweats (1)
Pain in the upper abdomen (1)
Palms of hands and soles of feet are both hot (2)*
Paralysis (1)
Ringing in the ears (1)
Sleeplessness with forgetfulness (1)
Weak loins and tibia (1)
Withering complexion (1)
Treatment principle: to water the liver and the kidneys yin
Treatment formula: *Jian-Ling-Tang*
Food cures: bird's nest, cheese, chicken egg, kidney bean, brown sugar, mussel, abalone, asparagus, chicken egg, cuttlefish, duck, duck

egg, white fungus, oyster, pork, royal jelly, chestnut, chicken liver, and pork kidneys

Uremia

1. Stomach energy upsurging syndrome ( )

Symptoms:
Dysphagia (3)
Dry vomiting (2)
Eating in the evening and vomiting in the morning (2)
Eating in the morning and vomiting in the evening (2)
Fatigue (1)
Hiccups in short sounds (3)
Nausea (1)
Sleepiness (1)
Upset stomach (3)
Vomiting of foods, watery sputum, or acidic and bitter water (1)
Vomiting right after eating (1)
Treatment principle: to harmonize the stomach and push down the upsurging stomach energy
Treatment formula: *Xiao-Ban-Xia-Jia-Fu-Ling-Tang*
Food cures: almond, areca nut, sugar beet, brake, buckwheat, common carp, cashew nut, coriander, loquat, malt, pea, black and white pepper, radish, rice bran, and sword bean

2. Kidneys yang deficiency syndrome ( )

Symptoms:
Cold feet or cold loins and legs (1)
Cold sensations in the genitals or the muscles (1)
Cough and panting (1)
Diarrhea before dawn (1)
Diarrhea with sticky and muddy stools (1)
Edema (1)
Fatigue (1)
Frequent urination at night (1)
Hair falling out easily (1)
Impotence (1)
Infertility (1)
Lack of appetite (1)
Pain in the loins (lumbago) (1)
Palpitations (1)
Panting (1)
Perspiration on the forehead (1)
Retention of urine (1)
Ringing in ears (1)
Shortness of breath (1)
Wheezing (1)
Treatment principle: to warm the kidneys yang and strengthen the true yin of the kidneys
Treatment formula: *Di-Huang-Yin-Zi*
Food cures: kidneys, lobster, sardine, shrimp, sparrow, clove, dill seed, fennel, pistachio nut, sparrow egg, crab apple, raspberry, and walnut

3. Spleen-kidneys deficiency syndrome ( )

Symptoms:
Diarrhea (3)
Difficult urination (2)
Dizziness (2)
Fatigue of the four limbs (3)
Insomnia (2)
Misty vision (2)
Palpitations (2)
Shortness of breath (2)
Yellowish complexion (2)
Treatment principle: to strengthen the spleen and the kidneys simultaneously
Treatment formula: *Ren-Shen-Yang-Ying-Tang*
Food cures: chicken egg yolk, common button mushroom, wheat bran, rice, beef, cherry, bird's nest, coconut meat, date, tofu,

mustard seed, sweet potato, red and black date, rock sugar, apple cucumber, carrot, chestnut, Irish potato, abalone, asparagus, chicken egg, white fungus, black sesame seed, beef kidneys, chicken liver, lobster, pork kidneys, raspberry, scallop, sea cucumber, shrimp, string bean, and walnut

CEREBROVASCULAR ACCIDENT

Cerebral Hemorrhage

1. Yang closure type (   )

Symptoms:
Both fists closed tightly (2)
Breathe heavily (4)*
Loud sputum sound like the sound of sawing (4)*
Neither urination nor bowel movement (4)*
Red complexion (3)*
Lockjaw (2)
Sudden fainting with complete unconsciousness (1)
Treatment principle: to wake up the patient by acupuncture or other forms of first aid
Treatment formula: Use *Kai-Guan-San* to open the lockjaw first, and then use 1 tablet of *Zhi-Bao-Dan* (crush into powder first) mixed with warm water and fresh ginger juice to administer to the patient through either the mouth or the nose; afterwards, use *Zhen-Gan-Xi-Feng-Tang*.

2. Yin closure type (   )

Symptoms:
Both fists closed tightly (3)
Cold limbs (4)*

Lockjaw (3)
Low but heavy sputum sound (4)*
Sudden fainting with complete unconsciousness (2)
Whitish or pale complexion (4)*
Treatment principle: to wake up the patient by acupuncture or other forms of first aid
Treatment formula: Use 1 tablet of *Su-He-Xiang-Wan* (crush into powder first) mixed with warm water and fresh ginger juice to administer to the patient through either the mouth or the nose; afterwards, use *Dao-Tan-Tang*.

3. Prolapse type (   )

Symptoms:
Both eyes are closed (3)
Cold limbs (2)
Hands are stretched after fainting (3)
Incontinence of urination (3)
Mouth remains open (3)
Perspiration (3)
Snoring (3)
Treatment principle: to wake up the patient by acupuncture or other forms of first aid
Treatment formula: Use the formula *Shen-Fu-Tang* (crush it into powder first) mixed with warm water and fresh ginger juice to administer to the patient through either the mouth or the nose; afterwards, use *Di-Huang-Yin-Zi*.

4. Aftereffects (   )

A. Hemiplegia (1)
Treatment principle: to tone the blood and energy simultaneously and to remove blood coagulations
Treatment formula: *Bu-Yang-Huan-Wu-Tang*

B. Speechlessness (1)

Treatment principle: to expel wind and remove sputum and to tone the yin and the yang

Treatment formula: *Di-Huang-Yin-Zi* for weaker patients, and *Tiao-Tan-Tang* for stronger patients

C. Wry eyes and mouth (1)

Treatment principle: to expel wind and remove sputum and to promote energy circulation

Treatment formula: *Qian-Zheng-San*

D. Incontinence of urination (1)

Treatment principle: to tone the middle region and strengthen energy and to strengthen the bladder and control urination

Treatment formula: *Bu-Zhong-Yi-Qi-Tang*

Cerebral Thrombosis (1)

Treatment principle: to expel wind and remove sputum and to activate the blood and promote blood circulation

Treatment formula: *Da-Qin-Jiao-Tang*

Subarachnoid Hemorrhage (1)

Treatment principle: to water the yin and cool the blood and to oppress the yang and stop the wind

Treatment formula: *Ling-Jiao-Gou-Teng-Tang*

NEUROSIS

Neurasthenia

1. Liver-fire upsurging syndrome ( )

Symptoms:
Acute dizziness (1)
Bleeding from stomach (1)

Dim eyes (1)
Dry sensations in the mouth (1)
Feeling hurried and quick-tempered (2)*
Getting angry easily (2)*
Headache that is severe (1)
Hiccups (1)
Many dreams (2)*
Nosebleed (1)
Pain in the upper abdomen (1)
Red eyes (1)
Ringing in ears (1)
Sleeplessness or sleep a lot (2)*
Vomiting of blood (1)
Yellowish-red urine (1)

Treatment principle: to sedate the liver-fire and nourish the heart

Treatment formula: *Long-Dan-Xie-Gan-Tang*

Food cures: spinach, chestnut, shepherd's purse, rye, black fungus, vinegar, abalone, asparagus, chicken egg, white fungus, pork, and royal jelly

2. Heart-spleen deficiency syndrome ( )

Symptoms:
Abdominal swelling (1)
Discharge of watery, thin stools (1)
Eating very little (1)
Fatigue (1)
Fatigue with lack of power (1)
Forgetfulness (1)
Impotence (1)
Nervous spirits (1)
Nervousness (1)
Night sweats (1)
Palpitations (1)
Shortness of breath (1)
Sleeplessness with many dreams (3)*
Underweight (1)
Wake up easily at night (3)*
Withering and yellowish complexion (1)

Treatment principle: to strengthen the spleen and energy and to tone the blood and nourish the heart

Treatment formula: *Gui-Pi-Tang*

Food cures: beef liver, chicken egg, cuttlefish, oyster, pork liver, sea cucumber, water spinach, longan nut, mandarin fish, apple cucumber, chestnut, horse bean, Job's-tears, Irish potato, rice, royal jelly, and yam

3. Heart-kidneys unable to communicate with each other syndrome or heart-kidneys yin deficiency syndrome ( )

Symptoms:

Deafness (1)

Dizziness (1)

Face becomes red when fatigued or working hard (1)

Feeling miserable (1)

Feeling miserable with love of darkness and dislike of light (1)

Forgetfulness (4)*

Light but periodic fever not unlike the tide (1)

Nervousness (1)

Night sweats (4)*

Palpitations (2)

Ringing in ears (1)

Sleeplessness with forgetfulness (1)

Sore loins and weak legs (1)

Treatment principle: to nourish the yin and clear internal heat and to promote communication between the heart and the kidneys

Treatment formula: *Liu-Wei-Di-Huang-Wan* with *Huang-Lian-E-Jiao-Tang*

Food cures: asparagus, abalone, chicken egg, white fungus, bog bean, wheat, banana, bamboo

shoot, bitter endive, oyster, royal jelly, and pork

Hysteria

1. Heart-spleen deficiency syndrome ( )

Symptoms:

Abdominal swelling (1)

Discharge of watery, thin stools (1)

Eating very little (1)

Fatigue (2)

Fatigue without power (1)

Forgetfulness (1)

Frequent yawning (3)*

Nervousness (1)

Night sweats (1)

Palpitations (1)

Sadness with a desire to cry (3)*

Shortness of breath (2)

Sleeplessness (2)

Withering and yellowish complexion (1)

Treatment principle: to tone the energy and blood simultaneously and to lubricate dryness and slow down progression of symptoms

Treatment formula: *Gan-Mai-Da-Zao-Tang*

Food cures: beef liver, chicken egg, cuttlefish, oyster, pork liver, sea cucumber, water spinach, longan nut, mandarin fish, apple cucumber, chestnut, horse bean, Job's-tears, Irish potato, rice, royal jelly, and yam

2. Liver energy congestion syndrome ( )

Symptoms:

Abdominal obstruction (1)

Abdominal pain (1)

Convulsions (1)

Feeling very depressed (3)*

Frequent sighing (3)*

Pain in the upper abdomen (2)
Premature menstrual periods (1)
Shortage of milk secretion after childbirth (1)
Stomachache (2)
Subjective sensations of objects in the throat (3)*
Vomiting of blood (1)
Whitish vaginal discharge (1)
Treatment principle: to relieve the liver energy congestion, transform sputum, and push down the upsurging energy
Treatment formula: *Ban-Xie-Hou-Pu-Tang*
Food cures: Brown sugar, garlic, turmeric, kumquat, beef, cherry, bird's nest, butterfish, chicken, coconut meat, date, tofu, mustard seed, sweet rice, goose meat, mutton, jackfruit, squash, sweet potato, red and black date, rice, rock sugar, caraway seed, spearmint, common button mushroom, oregano, red bean, ambergris, dill seed, sweet basil, and saffron

DEMENTIA, INCLUDING ALZHEIMER'S DISEASE

1. Spleen-sputum syndrome ( )

Symptoms:
Abundant saliva (?)
Being silent all day long (4)*
Bronchiectasis (1)
Loss of memory (4)*
Overweight, but eat only a small amount of food (1)
Poor appetite (1)
Slight fullness of the stomach (1)
Sudden crying and sudden laughing (4)*
Weakened limbs (2)

Treatment principle: to strengthen the spleen and remove sputum
Treatment formula: *Liu-Jun-Zi-Tang* or *Xi-Xin-Tang*
Food cures: bamboo shoot, crown daisy, date, fresh ginger, leaf or brown mustard, black and white pepper, white or yellow mustard seed, asparagus, and pear

2. Simultaneous occurrence of sputum congestion and blood coagulations syndrome ( )

Symptoms:
Alternating illogical talking and silence (2)*
Alternating silence and jumpiness (3)*
Chest pain (2)
Heavy sensations (1)
Insanity (2)
Lumpy spots in the body that do not shift (2)
Numbness (2)
Prickling and chronic pain in a fixed region that does not shift (2)
Symptoms get worse in cold weather and better in warm weather (2)
Unclear consciousness (2)
Treatment principle: to disperse the liver energy congestion and to transform blood coagulations and remove sputum
Treatment formula: *Chen Shi Yi Zhuan-Dai-Dan*
Food cures: bamboo shoot, crown daisy, date, fresh ginger, leaf or brown mustard, black and white pepper, white or yellow mustard seed, asparagus, and pear

3. Hot sputum syndrome ( )
Symptoms:
Asthma history (1)

143

Chronic dementia now getting worse
(4)*
Coma (1)
Cough (1)
Discharge of hard, yellow sputum in
lumps (1)
Discharge of sticky, turbid, and thin
stools (1)
Discharge of yellow, sticky sputum in
lumps (1)
Insanity (2)
Insomnia (3)
Stools with an extremely bad smell
(1)
Vomiting (1)
Wheezing (3)
Treatment principle: to clear hot
sputum
Treatment formula: *Wen-Dan-Tang*
Food cures: banana, bitter endive,
black fungus, salt, spinach,
strawberry, bamboo shoot,
cucumber, Job's-tears, laver, leaf
beet, mung bean, peppermint,
purslane, salt, cattail, agar, radish,
crown daisy, date, fresh ginger,
leaf or brown mustard, black and
white pepper, white or yellow
mustard seed, asparagus, and pear

4. Spleen-kidneys yang deficiency syndrome ( )

Symptoms:
Being silent all day or speechlessness
(2)*
Clear signs of aging (2)*
Cold hands and feet or cold loins (1)
Diarrhea before dawn (1)
Diarrhea with sticky and muddy
stools (1)
Edema that occurs all over the body
(1)
Fatigue (1)
Fear of cold (1)
Frequent urination in clear or white
streams (1)

Incontinence of urination and bowel
movement (2)*
Loss of memory (2)*
Paralysis of limbs (2)*
Slow movement (2)*
Sputum rumbling with panting (1)
Treatment principle: to warm the
kidneys and the spleen and to
transform sputum and remove
blood coagulations
Treatment formula: *Shen-Qi-Wan*
with *Er-Chen-Tang*
Food cures: air bladder of shark,
chicken, cayenne pepper, fennel,
nutmeg, black and white pepper,
prickly ash, mutton, sword bean,
white or yellow mustard, kidneys,
lobster, sardine, shrimp, sparrow,
clove, dill seed, pistachio nut,
sparrow egg, crab apple,
raspberry, and walnuts

5. Liver-kidneys yin deficiency syndrome ( )

Symptoms:
Dizziness (1)
Dry eyes or throat (1)
Explosive laughter and crying (2)*
Fatigue (1)
Headache with pain in the brow (1)
Hemiplegia (2)*
Loss of speech (2)*
Lumbago (1)
Night blindness (1)
Night sweats (1)
Pain in the upper abdomen (1)
Palms of hands and soles of feet are
both hot (1)
Poor memory (1)
Shaking of hands (2)*
Sleeplessness with forgetfulness (1)
Weak loins and tibia (1)
Treatment principle: to water the
yin and soften up the liver and to
transform blood coagulations and
stop the internal wind

Treatment formula: *Liu-Wei-Di-Huang-Wan* or *Sang-Nu-San-Jia-Tang*

Food cures: bird's nest, cheese, chicken egg, kidney bean, brown sugar, mussel, abalone, asparagus, chicken egg, cuttlefish, duck, duck egg, white fungus, oyster, pork, royal jelly, chestnut, chicken liver, and pork kidneys

6. Simultaneous energy congestion and blood coagulations syndrome (   )

Symptoms:
Abdominal swelling (2)
Being indifferent or pathetic emotionally (3)*
Congested chest (2)
Forgetfulness (2)
Hallucination (3)*
Love of sighing (1)
Lump in the abdomen that stays in the same region (1)
Slow response (3)*
Sudden fear and nervousness (3)*
Treatment principle: to activate the blood and transform coagulations and to promote energy circulation
Treatment formula: *Tao-Ren-Fu-Su-Fang*
Food cures: beef, cherry, bird's nest, butterfish, chicken, coconut meat, date, tofu, mustard seed, sweet rice, goose meat, mutton, jackfruit, squash, sweet potato, red and black date, rice, rock sugar, caraway seed, spearmint, common button mushroom, oregano, red bean, ambergris, dill seed, garlic, sweet basil, saffron, brown sugar, chestnut, eggplant, peach, black soybean, sturgeon, crab, distillers' grains, papaya, and saffron

ALLERGIES

Food Allergies

1. Liver offending the spleen syndrome (   )

Symptoms:
Abdominal enlargement (2)
Abdominal pain (2)
Abdominal rumbling (1)
Chronic diarrhea (2)
Diarrhea with watery stools often triggered by foods (5)*
Digestive breakdown often intensified by emotional upset (5)*
Fatigued spirits (1)
Hungry with no appetite (1)
Thirst with no desire for drink (1)
Treatment principle: to inhibit the liver and support the spleen and to regulate energy and dry up dampness
Treatment formula: *Tong-Xie-Yao-Fang* with *Ping-Wei-San*
Food cures: brown sugar, kumquat, mandarin orange, apple cucumber, bog bean, gold carp, carrot, chestnut, corncob, horse bean, hyacinth bean, Job's-tears, Irish potato, royal jelly, string bean, whitefish, and yam

2. Spleen-stomach deficiency syndrome (   )

Symptoms:
Abdominal pain (1)
Allergic to cold foods and greasy foods in particular (4)*
History of chronic enteritis, chronic gastritis, or chronic hepatitis (4)*
Diarrhea (1)
Dysentery alternating with very soft stools (4)*
Edema (1)
Falling of stomach (gastroptosis) (1)

Hiccups (1)
Plenty of saliva (1)
Rickets (1)
Stomachache (1)

Treatment principle: to strengthen the spleen and the stomach

Treatment formula: *Shen-Ling-Bai-Zhu-San*

Food cures: star anise, cayenne pepper, fresh ginger, chicken, clove, black and white pepper, apple cucumber, chestnut, ham, horse bean, Irish potato, rice, royal jelly, beef, red and black date, garlic, pistachio nut, barley, and rock sugar

3. Cold-dampness large-intestine syndrome ( )

Symptoms:
Abdominal pain (2)
Abdominal pain with abdominal rumbling (2)
Abdominal rumbling (2)
Clear and long streams of urine (1)
Cold hands and feet (1)
Congested chest (1)
Discharge of pure-white substances (4)*
Discharge of sticky, muddy stools not unlike goose dung (1)
Heavy sensations in the body (4)*
Poor appetite (2)

Treatment principle: to warm and transform cold and dampness

Treatment formula: *Wei-Ling-Tang*

Food cures: capers, cayenne pepper, fresh ginger, prickly ash, star anise, white or yellow mustard seed, white or yellow mustard, wine, chicken, clove, herring, nutmeg, and black and white pepper

4. Energy congestion syndrome ( )

Symptoms:
Abdominal pain (2)
Belching (1)
Chest and ribs discomfort (1)
Chest pain (2)
Constipation with a desire to empty the bowel (2)*
Discharge of stools like sheep dung (2)*
Pain in inner part of stomach with prickling sensation and swelling (1)
Pain in the upper abdomen (2)
Retention of urine (1)
Ringing in ears and deafness (1)
Stomachache (2)
Subjective sensation of lump in the throat (1)
Swallowing difficulty (1)
Swelling and congestion after eating (1)

Treatment principle: to promote energy circulation and disperse energy congestion

Treatment formula: *Liu-Mo-Yin* or *Wu-Mo-Yin-Zi*

Food cures: banana, bitter endive, black fungus, salt, spinach, strawberry, bamboo shoot, cucumber, Job's-tears, laver, leaf beet, mung bean, peppermint, purslane, salt, cattail, agar, radish, crown daisy, date, fresh ginger, leaf or brown mustard, black and white pepper, white or yellow mustard seed, asparagus, and pear

Environmental Allergies, Including Allergies Caused by Pollution, Plants, and Animals

Allergies of the Eyes, Including Spring Catarrh, Spring Conjunctivitis, and Other Allergic Reactions of the Eyes

1. Wind-heat syndrome ( )

Symptoms:
Burning sensation and uncomfortable dryness in the eyes (2)*
Coughing out blood (1)
Dizziness (1)
Headache (1)
Headache with dizziness (1)
Intolerable itch in the eyes (2)*
Intolerance of light in eyes with swelling and dislike of wind (1)
Muddy discharge from nose (1)
Nosebleed (1)
Pain in the eyes (2)*
Red eyes (2)*
Ringing in ears and deafness (1)
Tenesmus (1)
Thirst (1)
Toothache (1)
Yellow urine (1)
Yellowish discharge from the nose (1)
Treatment principle: to expel wind and activate the blood and to clear heat and nourish the blood
Treatment formula: *Xi-Gan-San*
Food cures: banana, bitter endive, black fungus, salt, spinach, strawberry, bamboo shoot, cucumber, Job's-tears, laver, leaf beet, mung bean, peppermint, purslane, spearmint, sweet basil, celery, coconut meat, and green onion

2. Wind-dampness-heat syndrome ( )

Symptoms:
Chronic backache (1)
Diarrhea (1)
Eczema (1)
Edema (1)
Eyes in dark-red color (3)*
Fever that becomes more severe in the afternoon (1)
Headache with heavy sensations in the head (1)
Itch in the eyes not very severe (3)*
Itchy sores (1)
Light swelling (1)
Pain in all the joints (2)
Pain shifting around with no fixed region (1)
Scant urine (1)
Whites of the eyes not very clear as if covered with a colloid substance (2)*
Treatment principle: to expel wind and clear heat and to remove dampness and stop itch
Treatment formula: *Xiao-Feng-San*
Food cures: peppermint, spearmint, sweet basil, celery, coconut meat, green onion, jellyfish skin, prickly ash, rice, adzuki bean, rosin, and tangerine

Allergies of the Nose, Including Hay Fever, Pollen Rhinitis, Allergic Rhinitis, and Other Allergic Reactions of the Nose

1. Lungs energy deficiency and cold syndrome ( )

Symptoms:
Breathing difficulty (1)
Common cold (1)
Copious, clear, and watery sputum (1)
Cough (1)

Excessive perspiration (1)
Fatigue (1)
Fear of cold (1)
Frequent sneezing (2)*
Impaired sense of smell (2)*
Light wheezing (1)
Low and weak voice (1)
Nasal congestion (2)*
Severe itch in the nose (2)*
Shortness of breath (1)
Smooth urination (1)
Too tired to talk (1)
Treatment principle: to warm and strengthen the lungs and to expel cold and drive out wind
Treatment formula: Wen-Fei-Zhi-Liu-Dan or Yu-Ping-Feng-San with Cang-Er-Zi-San
Food cures: cheese, Job's-tears, yam, grape, longan nuts, maltose, mandarin fish, Irish potato, sweet rice, apple cucumber, bog bean, gold carp, carrot, chestnut, ham, horse bean, hyacinth bean, royal jelly, string bean, whitefish, yam, red and black date, mutton, squash, and rock sugar

2. Spleen-lungs energy deficiency syndrome (   )

Symptoms:
Abdominal swelling (1)
Clear and white nasal discharge (3)*
Cough (1)
Coughing out and spitting of sputum and saliva (1)
Decreased appetite (1)
Decreased sense of smell (3)*
Diarrhea with sticky and muddy stools (1)
Discharge of copious, clear, watery sputum (1)
Eating only a little and with indigestion (1)
Fatigue of the four limbs (1)

Fatigue with lack of power (1)
Prolonged cough (1)
Rapid panting (1)
Shortness of breath (1)
Underweight and weak (2)
Treatment principle: to strengthen the spleen and to tone up the energy and the lungs
Treatment formula: Si-Jun-Zi-Tang with Shen-Ling-Bai-Zhu-San
Food cures: grape, longan nuts, maltose, mandarin fish, Irish potato, sweet rice, apple cucumber, bog bean, gold carp, carrot, chestnut, ham, horse bean, hyacinth bean, Job's-tears, royal jelly, string bean, whitefish, yam, red and black date, mutton, squash, rock sugar, chicken egg yolk, cheese, and bean

3. Kidneys yang deficiency syndrome (   )

Symptoms:
Allergies all year round (1)*
Cold feet or cold loins and legs (1)
Cold sensations in the genitals or the muscles (1)
Diarrhea before dawn (1)
Diarrhea with sticky and muddy stools (1)
Discharge of watery, thin stools (1)
Edema (1)
Fatigue (1)
Frequent urination at night (1)*
Frequent sneezing with clear nasal discharge (1)*
Impotence in men (1)
Infertility in women (1)
Lack of appetite (1)
Palpitations (1)
Panting (1)
Perspiration on the forehead (1)
Retention of urine (1)
Ringing in ears (1)

Shortness of breath (1)

Wheezing (1)

Treatment principle: to tone the lungs and warm the kidneys

Treatment formula: *Shen-Qi-Wan* or *Wen-Fei-Zhi-Liu-Dan*

Food cures: kidneys, lobster, sardine, shrimp, sparrow, clove, dill seed, fennel, pistachio nut, sparrow egg, crab apple, raspberry, and walnut

4. Kidneys yin deficiency syndrome ( )

Symptoms:

Allergies all year round (2)*

Cold hands and feet (1)

Cough with sputum containing blood or coughing out fresh blood (1)

Deafness (1)

Dizziness (1)

Dry sensations in the mouth particularly at night (1)

Dry throat (1)

Fatigue (1)

Feeling miserable and hurried, with fever (1)

Fever at night with burning sensations in internal organs (1)

Hot sensations in the middle of palms or soles of feet (1)

Night sweats (1)

Pain in the heels (1)

Pain in the loins (lumbago) (1)

Retention of urine (1)

Ringing in ears (1)

Sleeplessness (1)

Spots in front of the eyes (1)

Thirst (1)

Treatment principle: to water the kidneys yin

Treatment formula: *Zuo-Gui-Wan*

Food cures: abalone, asparagus, chicken egg, cuttlefish, duck, duck egg, white fungus, oyster, pork, royal jelly, chestnut, chicken liver, and pork kidneys

APPENDIX

Herbal Formulas

For each of the treatment formulas listed in this book, information is included here in the following two categories: the formula name and the ingredients.

Formula   This is the Romanization of the name of the formula; it is also the Chinese pronunciation of the name. The number within the brackets after the name of the formula is the reference number of the formula as shown in *An Encyclopedic Dictionary of Chinese Herbal Formulas,* which I compiled and which contains more than 4,000 formulas. Take the first formula as an example. *Ai-Fu-Nuan-Gong-Wan* is the Romanization of the name of this formula, and 0196i is its reference number. Following the reference number are the Chinese characters for the formula.

Ingredients   Each ingredient is written in the Romanization of the name of that herb, followed by its pharmaceutical name and standard dosage, and then by its dosage used in the particular formula. Take the first formula as an example. *Ai-ye* is the name of an herb used in this formula, its pharmaceutical name is *Folium Artemisiae Argyi,* 4-11 g is the standard daily dosage when this herb is decocted by itself for consumption, and 90 g is the amount of this herb used in this particular formula.

Instructions   For some of the formulas, special instructions are presented. If no special instructions are presented, the formula is to be used by decoction for single-day consumption. It is always wise to ask your herbalist for instructions to meet your needs.

Since each herbal formula is accompanied by its Chinese characters, any knowledgeable Chinese herbalist should be able to make the formula for you. If there are no Chinese herb shops in your area, write to Natural Chinese Herbs Information Resources, Box 236, 1857 West 4th Avenue, Vancouver, BC V6J 1M4, Canada.

1

Formula: *Ai-Fu-Nuan-Gong-Wan* (0196i)

艾附暖宫丸

Ingredients:
Ai-Ye-(Folium Artemisiae Argyi, 4 to 11 g), 90 g • *Bai-shao-yao (Radix Paeoniae Alba,* 5 to 11 g), 90 g • *Chuan-xiong (Rhizoma Ligustici Chuanxiong,* 2 to 6 g), 90 g • *Dang-gui (Radix Angelicae Sinensis,* 5 to 11 g), 90 g • *Huang-qi (Radix Astragali Seu Hedysari,* 5–40 g), 90 g • *Rou-gui (Cortex Cinnamomi,* 1 to 5 g), 15 g • *Shu-di-huang (Radix Rehmanniae Praeparatae,* 11 to 18 g), 30 g • *Wu-zhu-yu (Fructus Euodiae,* 2 to 7 g), 90 g • *Xiang-fu (Rhizoma Cyperi,* 5 to 11 g),

180 g • *Xu-Duan (Radix Dipsaci,* 5 to 11 g), 45 g

Instructions: Grind into powder to make tablets, and take 9 g of tablets twice daily.

2
Formula: *An-Gong-Niu-Huang-Wan (0286)*

安宮牛黃丸

Ingredients:
Bing-pian (Borneol, 0.2 to 0.3 g), 8 g • *Huang-lian (Rhizoma Coptidis,* 2 to 12 g), 30 g • *Huang-qin (Radix Scutellariae,* 4 to 15 g, 30 g • *Niu-huang (Calculus Bovis,* 0.2 to 0.5 g), 30 g • *She-xiang (Moschus,* 0.01 to 0.03 g), 8.30 g • *Xi-jiao (Cornu Rhinoceri,* 1 to 2 g), 30 g • *Xiong-huang (Realgar,* 0.3 to 1.5 g), 30 g • *Yu-jin (Radix Curcumae,* 4 to 11 g), 30 g • *Zhen-Zhu (Margarita,* 0.3 to 0.7 g), 15 g • *Zhi-zi(Fructus gardeniae,* 7 to 16 g), 30 g • *Zhu-sha (Cinnabaris,* 0.3 to 1 g), 30 g

3
Formula: *An-Shen-Ding-Zhi-Wan (0324)*

安神定志丸

Ingredients:
Chang-pu (Rhizoma Calami, 4 to 7 g), 3 g • *Fu-Ling (Poria,* 7 to 14 g), 12 g • *Fu-shen (Buyury,* with pine root, 11 to 15 g), 9 g • *Long-chi (Dens Draconis,* 11 to 18 g), 15 g • *Ren-shen (Radix Ginseng,* 1 to 35 g), 9 g • *Yuan-zhi (Radix Polygalae,* 4 to 11 g), 6 g

Instructions. Grind into powder, and take 2 g of powder each time, twice daily.

4
Formula: *Ba-Zhen-Tang (0182)*

八珍湯

Ingredients:
Bai-shao-yao (Radix Paeoniae Alba, 5 to 11 g), 12 g • *Bai-zhu (Rhizoma Atractylodis Macrocephalae,* 5 to 11 g), 10 g • *Chuan-xiong (Rhizoma Ligustici Chuanxiong,* 2 to 6 g), 6 g • *Dang-gui (Radix Angelicae Sinensis,* 5 to 11 g), 12 g • *Dang-shen (Radix Codonopsis Pilosulae,* 11 to 15 g), 10 g • *Fu-ling (Poria,* 7 to 14 g), 12 g • *Gan-cao (Radix Glycyrrhizae,* 2 to 11 g), 3 g • *Shu-di-huang (Radix Rehmanniae Praeparatae,* 11 to 18 g), 15 g

5
Formula: *Ba-Zhen-Yi-Mu-Tang (0872)*

八珍益母湯

Ingredients:
(Use equal quantities of all ingredients.)
Bai-shao-yao (Radix Paeoniae Alba, 5 to 11 g) • *Bai-zhu (Rhizoma Atractylodis Macrocephalae,* 5 to 11 g) • *Chuan-xiong (Rhizoma Ligustici Chuanxiong* 2 to 6) • *Dang-gui (Radix Angelicae Sinensis,* 5 to 11 g) • *Dang Shen (Radix Codonopsis Pilosulae,* 11 to 15 g) • *Fu-ling (Poria,* 7 to 14 g) • *Gan-cao (Radix Glycyrrhizae,* 2 to 11 g) • *Shu-di-huang (Radix Rehanniae Praeparatae,* 11 to 18 g) • *Yi-mu-cao (Herba Leonuri,* 11 to 36 g)

6
Formula: *Ba-Zheng-San (0349)*

八正散

Ingredients:
(Use equal quantities of all ingredients.)
Bian-xu (Herba Polygoni Avicularis, 5 to 11 g) • *Che-qian-zi (Semen Plantaginis,* 4 to 11 g) • *Da-huang (Radix Et Rhizoma Rhei,* 4 to 15 g) • *Gan-cao-shao (Fine Root Glycyrrhizae,* 2 to 5 g) • *Hua-shi (Talcum,* 11 to 15 g) • *Mu-tong (Caulis Aristolochiae,* 4 to 8 g) • *Qu-mai (Herba Dianthi,* 5 to 11 g) • *Zhi-zi (Fructus Gardeniae,* 7 to 16 g)

Instructions: Grind into powder, and take 6 to 8 g of powder each time.

7

Formula: *Bai-He-Gu-Jin-Tang* (0360)

百合固金湯

Ingredients:

Bai-he (Bulbus Lilii, 5 to 11 g), 15 g •
Chi-shao-yao (Radix Paeoniae Rubra, 5 to
11 g), 9 g • *Chuan-bei-mu* (Bulbus
Fritillariae Cirrhosae, 4 to 14 g), 6 g •
Dang-gui (Radix Angelicae Sinensis, 5 to
11 g), 9 g • *Gan-cao* (Radix Glycyrrhizae,
2 to 11 g), 3 g • *Jie-geng* (Radix Platycodi,
2 to 5 g), 6 g • *Mai-men-dong* (Radix
Ophiopogonis, 5 to 11 g), 6 g • *Sheng-di*
(Radix Rehamanniae, 14 to 35 g), 12 g •
Shu-di-huang (Radix Rehmanniae
Praeparatae, 11 to 18 g), 9 g • *Xuan-shen*
(Radix Scrophulariae, 7 to 35 g), 9 g

8

Formula: *Bai-Hu-Jia-Gui-Zhi-Tang* (0065A)

白虎加桂枝湯

Ingredients:

Gan-cao (Radix Glycyrrhizae, 2 to 11 g),
6 g • *Gui-zhi* (Ramulus Cinnamomi, 2 to
10 g), 6 g • *Jing-mi* (polished rice,
flexible quantity), 9 g • *Shi-gao* (Gypsum
Fibrosum, 10 to 70 g), 15–60 g • *Zhi-mu*
(Rhizoma Anemarrhenae, 4 to 15 g), 12 g

9

Formula: *Ban-Xia-Bai-Zhu-Tian-Ma-Tang*
(0122)

半夏白术天麻湯

Ingredients:

Bai-zhu (Rhizoma Atractylodis
Macrocephalae, 5 to 11 g), 12 g • *Ban-
xia, zhi-ban-xia* (Rhizoma Pinelliae, 4 to
12 g), 12 g • *Chen-pi* (Pericarpium
Papaveris, 4 to 11 g), 10 g • *Fu-ling*
(Poria, 7 to 14 g), 15 g • *Gan-cao* (Radix
Glycyrrhizae, 2 to 11 g), 3 g • *Tian-ma*
(Rhizoma Gastrodiae, 4 to 11 g), 10 g

10

Formula: *Ban-Xia-Hou-Pu-Tang* (0099)

半夏厚朴湯

Ingredients:

Ban-xia (Rhizoma Pinelliae, 4 to 12 g),
12 g • *Fu-ling* (Poria, 7 to 14 g), 12 g •
Hou-po (Cortex Magnoliae Officinalis, 4 to
11 g), 12 g • *Sheng-jiang* (Rhizoma
Zingiberis Recens, 4 to 10 g), 9 g • *Zi-su-
ye* (Folium Perillae, 5 to 10 g), 12 g

11

Formula: *Ban-Xia-Xie-Xin-Tang* (0105)

半夏瀉心湯

Ingredients:

Ban-xia (Rhizoma Pinelliae, 4 to 12 g),
15 g • *Da-zao* (Fructus Ziziphi Jujubae, 7
to 18 g), 9 g • *Gan-cao, zhi-gan-cao*
(Radix Glycyrrhizae, 2 to 11 g), 3 g •
Gan-jiang (Rhizoma Zingiberis, 3 to 7 g),
9 g • *Huang-lian* (Rhizoma Coptidis, 2 to
12 g), 6 g • *Huang-qin* (Radix
Scutellariae, 4 to 15 g), 9 g • *Ren-shen*
(Radix Ginseng, 1 to 35 g), 9 g

12

Formula: *Bao-He-Wan* (0074)

保和丸

Ingredients:

Ban-xia (Rhizoma Pinelliae, 4 to 12 g),
10 g • *Chen-pi* (Pericarpium Papaveris, 4
to 11 g), 10 g • *Fu-ling* (Poria, 7 to
14 g), 10 g • *Lai-fu-zi* (Semen Raphani, 5
to 11 g), 10 g • *Lian qiao* (Fructus
Forsythiae, 5 to 11 g), 10 g • *Shan-zha*
(Fructus Crataegi, 7 to 14 g), 10 g •
Shen-qu (Massa Medicata Fermentata, 7 to
15 g), 12 g

13

Formula: *Bei-Xie-Fen-Qing-Yin* (0358)

萆薢分清飲

Ingredients:
Bai-zhu (Rhizoma Atractylodis Macrocephalae, 5 to 11 g), 6 g • Bei-xie (Rhizoma Dioscoreae Bishie, 11 to 18 g), 24 g • Che-qian-Zi (Semen Plantaginis, 4 to 11 g), 12 g • Dan-shen (Radix Salviae Miltiorrhizae, 5 to 10 g), 6 g • Fu-ling (Poria, 7 to 14 g), 6 g • Huang-bai (Cortex Phellodendri, 4 to 15 g), 6 g • Lian-zi-xin (Plumula Nelumbinis, 2 to 4 g), 6 g • Shi-chang-pu (Rhizoma Acori Graminei, 2 to 5 g), 3 g

14
Formula: *Bu-Fei-Tang* (0043)

補肺湯

Ingredients:
Huang-qi (Radix Astragali Seu Hedysari, 5 to 40 g), 24 g • Ren-shen (Radix Ginseng, 1 to 35 g), 9 g • Sang-bai-pi (Cortex Mori Radicis, 5 to 11 g), 12 g • Shu-di-huang (Radix Rehmanniae Praeparatae, 11 to 18 g), 24 g • Wu-wei-zi (Fructus Schisandrae, 2 to 4 g), 6 g • Zi-wan (Radix Asteris, 5 to 11 g), 9 g

15
Formula: *Bu-Huan-Jin-Zheng-Qi-San* (0117D)

不換金正氣散

Ingredients:
Ban-xia (rhizoma Pinelliae, 4 to 12 g), 10 g • Cang-zhu (Rhzoma Atractylodis Macrocephalae, 4 to 11 g), 10 g • Chen-pi (Pericarpium Papaveris, 4 to 11 g), 10 g • Gan-cao (Radix Glycyrrhizae, 2 to 11 g), 3 g • Hou-po (Cortex Magnoliae Officinalis, 4 to 11 g), 10 g • Huo-xiang (Herba Agastachis, 5 to 11 g), 10 g

16
Formula: *Bu-Xin-Dan* (0297)

補心丹

Ingredients:
Bai-zi-ren (Semen Biotae, 4 to 11 g), 30 g • Dan-shen (Radix Salviae Miltiorrhizae, 5 to 10 g), 15 g • Dang-gui (Radix Angelicae Sinensis, 5 to 11 g), 21 g • Fu-ling (Poria, 7 to 14 g), 12 g • Jie-geng (Radix Platycodi, 2 to 5 g), 9 g • Mai-men-Dong (Radix Ophiopogonis, 5 to 11 g), 9 g • Ren-shen (Radix Ginseng, 1 to 35 g), 9 g • Sheng-di (Radix Rehmanniae), 14 to 35 g), 30 g • Suan-zao-Ren (Semen Ziziphi Spinosae, 7 to 18 g), 30 g • Tian-dong (Radix Asparagi, 7 to 14 g), 9 g • Wu-wei-zi (Fructus Schisandrae, 2 to 4 g), 9g • Xuan-shen (Radix Scrophulariae, 7 to 35 g), 12 g • Yuan-zhi (Radix Polygalae, 4 to 11 g), 9 g

Instructions: Grind into powder to make tablets, and take 9 to 15 g of tablets each time.

17
Formula: *Bu-Yang-Huan-Wu-Tang* (0212)

補陽還五湯

Ingredients:
Chi-shao-yao (Radix Paeoniae Rubra, 5 to 11 g), 6 g • Chuan-xiong (Rhizoma Ligustici Chuanxiong, 2 to 6 g), 3 g • Dang-gui (Radix Angelicae Sinensis, 5 to 11 g), 6 g • Di-long (Lumbricus, 5 to 11 g), 3 g • Hong-hua (Flos Carthami, 4 to 7 g), 3 g • Huang-qi (Radix Astragali Seu Hedysari, 5 to 40 g), 120 g • Tao-ren (Semen Persicae, 5 to 11 g), 3 g

18
Formula: *Bu-Zhong-Yi-Qi-Tang* (0084)

補中益氣湯

Ingredients:
Bai-zhu (Rhizoma Atractylodis Macrocephalae, 5 to 11 g), 10 g • Chai-hu (Radix Bupleuri, 4 to 16 g), 6 g • Chen-pi (Pericarpium Papaveris, 4 to 11 g), 9 g • Dang-gui (Radix Angelicae Sinensis, 5 to 11 g), 10 g • Dang-shen (Radix Codonopsis Pilosulae, 11 to 15 g), 15 g • Gan-cao (Radix Glycyrrhizae, 2 to 11 g), 6 g • Huang-qi (Radix Astragali Seu Hedysari, 5 to 40 g), 24 g • Sheng-ma (Thizoma Cimicifugae, 3 to 10 g), 6 g

19

Formula: *Cang-Er-Zi-San* (0563)

蒼耳子散

Ingredients:
Bai-zhi (Radix Angelicae Dahuricae, 4 to 10 g), 3 g • *Bo-he* (Herba Menthae, 3 to 10 g), 6 g • *Cang-er-zi* (Fructus Xanthii, 4 to 11 g), 9 g • *Xin-yi* (Flos Magnoliae, 4 to 10 g), 6 g

20

Formula: *Chai-Hu-Shu-Gan-San* (0230A)

柴胡疏肝散

Ingredients:
Bai-shao-yao (Radix Paeoniae Alba, 5 to 11 g), 24 G • *Chai-hu* (Radix Bupleuri, 4 to 16 g), 9 g • *Chuan-xiong* (Rhizoma Ligustici Chuanxiong, 2 to 6 g), 6 g • *Gan-cao* (Radix Glycyrrhizae, 2 to 11 g), 6 g • *Gan-jiang* (Rhizoma Zingiberis, 3 to 7 g), g • *Xiang-fu* (Rhizoma Cyperi, 5 to 11 g), 12 g • *Zhi-qiao* (Fructus Auranth, 4 to 11 g), 9 g • *Zhi-zi* (Fructus Gardeniae, 7 to 16 g), g

21

Formula: *Chen-Shi-Yi-Zhuan-Dai-Dan* (3358)

陳氏鐸轉呆丹

Ingredients:
Bai-shao-yao (Radix Paeoniae Alba, 5 to 11 g), 8 g • *Ban-xia* (Rhizoma Pinelliae, 4 to 12 g), 6 g • *Chai-hu* (Radix Bupleuri, 4 to 16 g), 7 g • *Chen-pi* (Pericarpium Citri Reticulatae, 4 to 11 g), 6 g • *Dan-shen* (Radix Salviae Miltiorrhizae, 5 to 10 g), 6 g • Dang-gui (Radix Angelicae Sinensis, 5 to 11 g), 7 g • *Dang-shen* (Radix Codonopsis Pilosulae, 11 to 15 g), 6 g • *Fu-shen* (Buyury with pine root, 11 to 15 g), 6 g • *Gan-cao* (Radix Glycyrrhizae, 2 to 11 g), 5 g • *Mai-men-Dong* (Radix Ophiopogonis, 5 to 11 g), 6 g • *Shen-qu* (Massa Medicata Fermentata, 7 to 15 g), 8 g • *Shi-chang-pu* Rhizoma Acori Graminei, 2 to 5 g), 5 g • *Suan-zao-ren* (Semen Ziziphi Spinosae, 7 to 18 g), 8 g • *Tao-ren* (Semen Persicae, 5 to 11 g), 6 g • *Tian-hua-fen* (Radix Trichosanthis, 10 to 14 g), 10 g • *Xiang-fu* (Rhizoma Cyperi, 5 to 11 g), 6 g

22

Formula: *Chi-Xiao-Dou-Dang-Gui-San* (0571)

赤小豆當歸散

Ingredients:
Chi-xioa-dou (Semen Phaseoli, 11 to 18 g), 30 g • *Dang-gui* (Radix Angelicae Sinensis, 5 to 11 g), 15 g

23

Formula: *Chuan-Xiong-Cha-Tiao-San* (0011)

川芎茶調散

Ingredients:
Bai-zhi (Radix Angelicae Dahuricae, 4 to 10 g), 6 g • *Bo-he* (Herba Menthae, 3 to 10 g), 3 g • *Chuan-xiong* (Rhizoma Ligustici Chuanxiong, 2 to 6 g), 12 g • *Fang-feng* (Radix Ledebouriellae, 5 to 10 g), 6 g • *Gan-cao* (Radix Glycyrrhizae, 2 to 11 g), 6 g • *Jing-jie* (Herba Schizonepetae, 5 to 10 g), 12 g • *Qiang-huo* (Rhizoma Seu Radix Notopterygii Notopterygii, 4 to 10 g), 6 g • *Xi-xin* (Herba Asari, 1 to 4 g), 3 g

24

Formula: *Da-Bu-Yin-Wan* (0273)

大補陰丸

Ingredients:
Gui-ban (Plastrum Testudinis, 11 to 30 g), 180 g • *Huang-bai* (Cortex Phellodendri, 4 to 15 g), 120 g • *Shu-di-huang* (Radix Rehmanniae Praeparatae, 11 to 18 g), 180 g • *Zhi-mu* (Rhizoma Anemarrhenae, 4 to 15 g), 120 g

Instructions: Grind into powder and make tablets. Take six to nine tablets twice daily; if decoction is done, reduce dosages.

25
Formula: Da-Bu-Yuan-Jian (0399)

大補元煎

Ingredients:

Dang-gui (Radix Angelicae Sinensis, 5 to 11 g), 9 g • Du-zhong (Cortex Eucommiae, 7 to 11 g), 9 g • Gan-cao (Radix Glycyrrhizae, 2 to 11 g), 6 g • Gou-qi-zi (Fructus Lych, 5 to 11 g), 9 g • Ren-shen (Radix Ginseng, 1 to 35 g), 9 g • Shan-yao (Rhizoma Dioscoreae, 10 to 20 g), 9 g • Shan-zhu-yu (Fructus Corni, 5 to 11 g), 9 g • Shu-di-huang (Radix Rehmanniae Praeparatae, 11 to 18 g), 15 g

26
Formula: Da-Chai-Hu-Tang (0256)

大柴胡湯

Ingredients:

Bai-shao-Yao (Radix Paeoniae Alba, 5 to 11 g), 30 g • Ban-xia (Rhizoma Pinelliae, 4 to 12 g), 15 g • Chai-hu (Radix Bupleuri, 4 to 16 g), 21 g • Da-huang (Radix Et Rhizoma Rhei, 4 to 15 g), 15 g • Da-zao (Fructus Ziziphi Jujubae, 7 to 18 g), four dates • Huang-qin (Radix Scutellariae, 4 to 15 g), 15 g • Sheng-jiang (Rhizoma Zingiberis Recens, 4 to 10 g), 9 g • Zhi-shi (Fructus Aurantii Immaturus, 4 to 7 g), 6 g

27
Formula: Da-Cheng-Qi-Tang (0146)

大承氣湯

Ingredients:

Da-huang (Radix Et Rhizoma Rhei, 4 to 15 g), 12 g • Hou-po (Cortex Magnoliae Officinalis, 4 to 11 g), 15 g • Pu-xiao (Mirabilitum Depuratum, 5 to 11 g), 12 g

• *Zhi-shi (Fructus Aurantii Immaturus, 4 to 7 g), 10 g*

28
Formula: Da-Ding-Feng-Zhu (0247)

大定風珠

Ingredients:

Bai-shao-yao (Radix Paeoniae Alba, 5 to 11 g), 18 g • Bie-jia (Carapax Trionycis, 11 to 18 g), 12 g • E-jiao (Colla Corii Asini, 5 to 11 g), 9 g • Gan-cao (Radix Glycyrrhizae, 2 to 11 g), 12 g • Gui-ban (Plastrum Testudinis, 11 to 30 g), 12 g • Huo-ma-Ren (Fructus Cannabis, 11 to 17 g), 6 g • Ji-zi-huang (Chicken egg yolk, flexible g), two eggs • Mai-men-dong (Radix Ophiopogonis, 5 to 11 g), 18 g • Mu-li (Concha Ostrae, 11 to 35 g), 12 g • Sheng-di (Radix Rehmanniae, 14 to 35 g), 18 g • Wu-wei-zi (Fructus Schisandrae, 2 to 4 g), 6 g

29
Formula: Da-Qin-Jiao-Tang (0279)

大秦艽湯

Ingredients:

Bai-shao-yao (Radix Paeoniae Alba, 5 to 11 g), 18 g • Bai-zhi (Radix Angelicae Dahuricae, 4 to 10 g), 9 g • Bai-zhu (Rhizoma Atractylodis Macrocephalae, 5 to 11 g), 12 g • Chuan-xiong (Rhizoma Ligustici Chuanxiong, 2 to 6), 9 g • Dang-gui (Radix Angelicae Sinensis, 5 to 11 g), 9 g • Du-huo (Radix Angelicae Pubescentis, 2 to 5 g), 12 g • Fang-feng (Radix Ledebouriellae, 5 to 10 g), 9g • Fu-ling (Poria, 7 to 14 g), 12 g • Gan-cao (Radix Glycyrrhizae, 2 to 11 g), 6 g • Huang-qin (Radix Scutellariae, 4 to 15 g), 9 g • Qiang-Huo (Rhizoma Seu Radix Notopterygii Notopterygh, 4 to 10 g), 9 g • Qin-jiao (Radix Gentianae Macrophyllae, 4 to 11 g), 15 g • Sheng-di (Radix Rehmanniae, 14 to 35 g), 12 g • Shi-gao (Gypsum Fibrosum, 10 to 70 g), 18 g • Shu-di-huang (Radix Rehmannice

Praeparatae, 11 to 18 g), 12 g • Xi-xin
(Herba Asari, 1 to 4 g), 6 g

30
Formula: Da-Yuan-Yin (0257)

達原飲

Ingredients:
Bai-shao-Yao (Radix Paeoniae Alba, 5 to
11 g), 9 g • Bing-lang (Semen Areca, 4 to
11 g), 12 g • Cao-guo (Fructus Tsaoko, 2
to 5 g), 3 g • Gan-cao (Radix
Glycyrrhizae, 2 to 11 g), 3 g • Hou-po
(Cortex Magnoliae Officinalis, 4 to 11 g),
9 g • Huang-qin (Radix Scutellariae, 4 to
15 g), 12 g • Zhi-mu (Rhizoma
Anemarrhenae, 4 to 15 g), 12 g

31
Formula: Dai-Di-Dang-Wan (0982)

代抵當丸

Ingredients:
Chuan-shan-jia (Squama Manitis, 5 to
11 g), 30 g • Da-huang (Radix Et
Rhizoma Rhei, 4 to 15 g), 120 g • Dang-
gui (Radix Angelicae Sinensis, 5 to 11 g),
30 g • Mang-xiao (Natrii Sulfas, 4 to
11 g), 30 g • Rou-gui (Cortex Cinnamomi,
1 to 5 g), 15 g • Sheng-di (Radix
Rehmanniae, 14 to 35 g), 30 g • Tao-ren
(Semen Persicae, 5 to 11 g), 30 g
Instructions: Grind into powder to make
tablets, and take 9 g of tablets twice
daily.

32
Formula: Dan-Tian-Jiang-Zhi-Wan (3359)

丹田降脂丸

Ingredients:
Chuan-xiong (Rhizoma Ligustici
Chuanxiong, 2 to 6 g), 6 g • Dan-shen
(Radix Salviae Miltiorrhizae, 5 to 10 g),
10 g • Dang-gui (Radix Angelicae Sinensis,
5 to 11 g), 11 g • He-shou-Wu (Radix
Polygoni Multiflori, 11 to 15 g), 15 g •

Huang-jing (Rhizoma Polygonati, 11 to
15 g), 15 g • Ren-shen (Radix Ginseng, 1
to 35 g), 35 g • San-qi (Radix
Notoginseng, 2 to 10 g), 10 g • Ze-xie
(Rhizoma Alismatis, 7 to 14 g), 14 g

33
Formula: Dan-Zhi-Xiao-Yao-San (0229A)

丹梔逍遙散

Ingredients:
Bai-shao-yao (Radix Paeoniae Alba, 5 to
11 g), 30 g • Bai-zhu (Rhizoma
Atractylodis Macrocephalae, 5 to 11 g), 9 g
• Chai-hu (Radix Bupleuri, 4 to 16 g), 9 g
• Dang-gui (RAdix Angelicae Sinensis, 5 to
11 g), 9 g • Fu-ling (Poria, 7 to 14 g),
15 g • Gan-cao (Radix Glycyrrhizae, 2 to
11 g), 6 g • Mu-dan-pi (Cortex Moutan
Radicis, 5 to 11 g), g • Zhi-zi (Fructus
Gardeniae, 7 to 16 g), g

34
Formula: Dang-Gui-Jian-Zhong-Tang
(0064C)

當歸建中湯

Ingredients:
Chi-shao-yao (Radix Paeoniae Rubra, 5 to
11 g), 30 g • Da-zao (Fructus Ziziphi
Jujubae, 7 to 18 g), 10 g • Dang-gui
(Radix Angelicae Sinensis, 5 to 11 g), 20 g
• Gan-cao (Radix Glycyrrhizae, 2 to 11 g),
10 g • Gui-zhi (Ramulus Cinnamomi, 2 to
10 g), 15 g • Sheng-jiang (Rhizoma
Zingiberis Recens, 4 to 10 g), 15 g • Yi-
tang (Saccharum Granorum, 30 to 60 g),
60 g

35
Formula: Dang-Gui-Long-Hui-Wan (0189)

當歸芦荟丸

Ingredients:
Da-huang (Radix Et Rhizoma Rhei, 4 to
15 g), 15 g • Dang-gui (Radix Angelicae
Sinensis, 5 to 11 g), 30 g • Huang-bai

(Cortex Phellodendri, 4 to 15 g), 30 g •
Huang-lian (Rhizoma Coptidis, 2 to 12 g),
30 g • Huang-qin (Radix Scutellariae, 4 to
15 g), 30 g • Long-dan (Radix Gentianae,
7 to 10 g), 30 g • Lu-hui (Aloe, 2 to 5 g),
15 g • Mu-xiang (Radix
Aucklandiae/Radix Saussureae, 2 to 6 g),
6 g • Qing-dai (Indigo Naturalis, 2 to
4 g), 15 g • She-xiang (Moschus, 0.01 to
0.03 g), 1.5 g • Zhi-zi (Fructus
Gardeniae, 7 to 16 g), 30 g

Instructions: Grind into powder, and
take 5 g of powder each time, twice
daily.

36
Formula: Dao-Chi-Cheng-Qi-Tang (1049)

導赤承氣湯

Ingredients:
(Use equal quantities of all ingredients.)
Chi-shao-yao (Radix Paeoniae Rubra, 5 to
11 g) • Da-huang (Radix Et Rhizoma Rhei,
4 to 15 g) • Huang-bai (Cortex
Phellodendri, 4 to 15 g) • Huang-lian
(Rhizoma Coptidis, 2 to 12 g) • Mang-
xiao (Natrii Sulfas/Mirabilitum
Depuratum, 4 to 11 g) • Sheng-di (Radix
Rehmanniae, 14 to 35 g)

Instructions: Grind into powder, and
take 6 g of powder each time, twice
daily.

37
Formula: Dao-Chi-San (0357)

導赤散

Ingredients:
Gan-cao shao (Fine Root Glycyrrhizae, 2 to
5 g), 6 g • Mu-tong (Caulis Aristolochiae,
4 to 8 g), 12 g • Sheng-di (Radix
Rehmanniae, 14 to 35 g), 24 g • Zhu-ye
(Folium Bambusae, 4 to 20 g), 6 g

Instructions: Decoct the herbs by adding
Deng-Xin-Cao (Medulla Junci, 2 to
3 g), 6 g

38
Formula: Dao-Tan-Tang (0123)

導痰湯

Ingredients:
Ban-xia (Rhizoma Pinelliae, 4 to 12 g),
15 g • Chen-pi Pericarpium Papaveris, 4
to 11 g), 10 g • Fu-ling (Poria, 7 to
14 g), 12 g • Gan-cao (Radix
Glycyrrhizae, 2 to 11 g), 3 g • Sheng-jiang
(Rhizoma Zingiberis Recens, 4 to 10 g),
10 g • Tian-nan-xing (Rhizoma
Arisaematis, 2.5 to 5 g), 12 g • Zhi-qiao
(Fructus Aurantii, 4 to 11 g), 10 g

39
Formula: De-Sheng-Dan (1841)

得生丹

Ingredients:
Bai-shao-yao (Radix Paeoniae Alba, 5 to
11 g), 80 g • Chai-hu (Radix Bupleuri, 4
to 16 g), 30 g • Dang-gui (Radix
Angelicae Sinensis, 5 to 11 g), 80 g • Mu-
xiang (Radix Aucklandize, 6 g), 30 g •
Qiang-huo (Rhizoma Seu Radix
Notopterygii, 4 to 10 g), 30 g • Yi-mu-cao
(Herba Leonuri, 11 to 36 g), 320 g

Instructions: Grind into powder to make
tablets with honey, and take 10 g of
tablets twice daily.

40
Formula: Di-Huang-Yin-Zi (0532)

地黃飲子

Ingredients:
Gan-cao (Radix Glycyrrhizae, 2 to 11 g),
5 g • Huang-qi (Radix Astragali seu
Hedysari, 5 to 40 g), 20 g • Mai-men-
dong (Radix Ophiopogonis, 5 to 11 g), 5 g
• Pi-pa-ye (Folium Eriobotryae, 5 to 11 g),
5 g • Ren-shen (Radix Ginseng, 1 to 35 g),
20 g • Sheng-di (Radix Rehmanniae, 14 to
35 g), 25 g • Shi-hu (Herba Dendrobii, 7
to 14 g), 10 g • Shu-di-huang (Radix
Rehmanniae Praeparatae, 11 to 18 g), 15 g

• *Tian-dong (Radix Asparagi, 7 to 14 g),* 10 g • *Ze-xie (Rhizoma Alismatis, 7 to 14 g),* 10 g • *Zhi-qiao (Fructus Aurantii, 4 to 11 g),* 5 g

41

Formula: *Di-Tan-Tang (0293)*

滌痰湯

Ingredients:

Ban-xia (Rhizoma Pinelliae, 4 to 12 g), 15 g • *Chang-pu (Rhizoma Calami, 4 to 7 g),* 6 g • *Chen-pi (Pericarpium Papaveris, 4 to 11 g),* 9 g • *Dan-nan-xing (Arisaema Cum Bile, 4 to 8 g),* 12 g • *Fu-ling (Poria, 7 to 14 g),* 12 g • *Gan-cao (Radix Glycyrrhizae, 2 to 11 g),* 3 g • *Ren-shen (Radix Ginseng, 1 to 35 g),* 9 g • *Zhi-shi (Fructus Aurantii Immaturus, 4 to 7 g),* 9 g • *Zhu-ru (Caulis Bambusae in Taeniam, 5 to 11 g),* 15 g

42

Formula: *Ding-Xian-Wan (0592)*

定癎丸

Ingredients:

Ban-xia (Rhizoma Pinelliae, 4 to 12 g), 30 g • *Chang-pu (Rhizoma Calami, 4 to 7 g),* 15 g • *Chen-pi (Pericarpium Citri Reticulatae Viride, 4 to 11 g),* 21 g • *Chuan-bei-mu (Bulbus Fritillariae Thunbergii Cirrhosae, 4 to 14 g),* 21 g • *Dan-nan-xing (Arisaema Cum Bile, 4 to 8 g),* 15 g • *Dan-shen (Radix Salviae Miltiorrhizae, 5 to 10 g),* 60 g • *Fu-ling (Poria, 7 to 14 g),* 30 g • *Fu-shen (Buyury with pine root, 11 to 15 g),* 30 g • *Gan-cao (Radix Glycyrrhizae, 2 to 11 g),* 21 g • *Hu-po (Succinum, 1 to 2 g),* 15 g • *Jiang-can (Bombyx Batryticatus, 5 to 11 g),* 15 g • *Mai-men-dong (Radix Ophiopogonis, 5 to 11 g),* 60 g • *Quan-xie (Scorpio, 2 to 5 g),* 15 g • *Sheng-jiang (Rhizoma Zingiberis Recens, 4 to 10 g),* 10 g • *Tian-ma (Rhizoma Gastrodiae, 4 to 11 g),* 30 g • *Yuan-zhi (Radix Polygalae, 4 to 11 g),* 21 g • *Zhu-li (Bamboo Liquid 30 to 60 g),* 10 g • *Zhu-sha (Cinnabaris, 0.3 to 1 g),* 15 g

Instructions: Grind into powder, and take 9 g of powder twice daily.

43

Formula: *Ding-Xiang-Shi-Di-Tang (0092)*

丁香柿蒂湯

Ingredients:

Ding-xiang (Flos Caryophylli, 1 to 4 g), 10 g • *Ren-shen (Radix Ginseng, 1 to 35 g),* 10 g • *Sheng-jiang (Rhizoma Zingiberis Recens, 4 to 10 g),* 12 g • *Shi-di (Calyx Kaki, 5 to 11 g),* 10 g

44

Formula: *Ding-Zhi-Wan (0306)*

定志丸

Ingredients:

Fu-ling (Poria, 7 to 14 g), 30 g • *Ren-shen (Radix Ginseng, 1 to 35 g),* 30 g • *Shi-chang-pu (Rhizoma Acori Graminei, 2 to 5 g),* 60 g • *Yuan-zhi (Radix Polygalae, 4 to 11 g),* 60 g

Instructions: Grind into powder, and take 6 g of powder each time; you may also decoct.

45

Formula: *Du-Huo-Ji-Sheng-Tang (0278)*

獨活寄生湯

Ingredients:

Chi-shao-yao (Radix Paeoniae Rubra, 5 to 11 g), 30 g • *Chuan-xiong (Rhizoma Ligustici Chuanxiong, 2 to 6 g),* 9 g • *Dang-gui (Radix Angelicae Sinensis, 5 to 11 g),* 9 g • *Du-huo (Radix Angelicae Pubescentis, 2 to 5 g),* 15 g • *Du-zhong (Cortex Eucommiae, 7 to 11 g),* 15 g • *Fang-feng (Radix Ledebouriellae, 5 to 10 g),* 9 g • *Fu-ling (Poria, 7 to 14 g),* 12 g • *Gan-cao (Radix Glycyrrhizae, 2 to 11 g),* 3 g • *Gan-di (Dried Radix Rehmanniae, 11 to 18 g),* 18 g • *Niu-xi (Radix Achyranthis Bidentatae, 5 to 11 g),* 15 g • *Qin-jiao (Radix Gentianae*

Macrophyllae, 4 to 11 g), 10 g • Ren-shen (Radix Ginseng, 1 to 35 g), 12 g • Rou-gui (Cortex Cinnamomi, 1 to 5 g), 9 g • Sang-ji-sheng (Ramulus Loranthi, 11 to 18 g), 24 g • Xi-xin (Herba Asari, 1 to 4 g), 6 g

46
Formula: *Er-Chen-Tang* (0121)

二陳湯

Ingredients:
Ban-xia (Rhizoma Pinelliae, 4 to 12 g), 15 g • Chen-pi (Pericarpium Papaveris, 4 to 11 g), 10 g • Fu-ling (Poria, 7 to 14 g), 15 g • Gan-cao (Radix Glycyrrhizae, 2 to 11 g), 3 g

47
Formula: *Er-Long-Zuo-Zi-Wan* (0327D)

耳聾左慈丸

Ingredients:
Ci-shi (Magnetitum, 11 to 35 g), 90 g • Fu-ling (Poria, 7 to 14 g), 90 g • Mu-dan-pi (Cortex Moutan Radicis, 5 to 11 g), 90 g • Shan-yao (Rhizoma Dioscoreae, 10 to 20 g), 120 g • Shan-zhu-yu (Fructus Corni, 5 to 11 g), 120 g • Shi-chang-pu (Rhizoma Acori Graminei, 2 to 5 g), 90 g • Shu-di-huang (Radix Rehmanniae Praeparatae, 11 to 18 g), 240 g • Wu-wei-zi (Fructus Schisandrae, 2 to 4 g), 90 g • Ze-Xie (Rhizoma Alismatis, 7 to 14 g), 90 g
Instructions: Grind into powder to make tablets, and take three tablets or 9 g two to three times daily.

48
Formula: *Er-Mu-San* (0366)

二母散

Ingredients:
(Use equal quantities of ingredients.)
Zhe-bei-mu (Bulbus Fritillariae Thunbergii, 5 to 11 g) • Zhi-mu (Rhizoma Anemarrhenae, 4 to 15 g)

Instructions: Grind into powder, and take 6 g of powder twice daily.

49
Formula: *Er-Yin-Jian* (0860)

二陰煎

Ingredients:
Deng-xin-cao (Medulla Junci, 2 to 3 g), 30 g • Fu-ling (Poria, 7 to 14 g), 12 g • Gan-cao (Radix Glycyrrhizae, 2 to 11 g), 10 g • Huang-lian (Rhizoma Coptidis, 2 to 12 g), 9 g • Mai-men dong (Radix Ophiopogonis, 5 to 11 g), 12 g • Mu-tong (Caulis Aristolochiae, 4 to 8 g), 9 g • Sheng-di (Radix Rehmanniae, 14 to 35 g), 12 g • Suan-zao-ren (Semen Ziziphi Spinosae, 7 to 18 g), 18 g • Xuan-shen (Radix Scrophulariae, 7 to 35 g), 10 g • Zhu-ye (Folium Bambusae, 4 to 20 g), 6 g

50
Formula: *Fang-Feng-Tang* (0535)

防風湯

Ingredients:
Dang-gui (Radix Angelicae Sinensis, 5 to 11 g), 6 g • Fang-feng (Radix Ledebouriellae, 5 to 10 g), 6 g • Fu-ling (Poria, 7 to 14 g), 6 g • Gan-cao (Radix Glycyrrhizae, 2 to 11 g), 3 g • Ge-gen (Radix Puerariae, 4 to 20 g), 9 g • Gui-zhi (Ramulus Cinnamomi, 2 to 10 g), 3 g • Huang-qin (Radix Scutellariae, 4 to 15 g), 9 g • Qiang-huo (Rhizoma Seu Radix Notopterygii, 4 to 10 g), 3 g • Qin-Jiao (Radix Gentianae Macrophyllae, 4 to 11 g), 9 g • Xing-Ren (Semen Armeniacae Amarae, 5 to 11 g), 6 g

51
Formula: *Fang-Feng-Tong-Sheng-San* (0536)

防風通聖散

Ingredients:
Bai-shao-yao (Radix Paeoniae Alba, 5 to 11 g), 15 g • Bai-zhu (Rhizoma

Atractylodis Macrocephalae, 5 to 11 g),
15 g • Bo-he (Herba Menthae, 3 to 10 g),
15 g • Chuan-xiong (Rhizoma Ligustici
Chuanxiong, 2 to 6 g), 15 g • Da-huang
(Radix Et Rhizoma Rhei, 4 to 15 g), 15 g
• Dang-gui (Radix Angelicae Sinensis, 5 to
11 g), 15 g • Fang-feng (Radix
Ledebouriellae, 5 to 10 g), 15 g • Gan-cao
(Radix Glycyrrhizae, 2 to 11 g), 60 g •
Hua-shi (Talcum, 11 to 15 g), 90 g •
Huang-qin (Radix Scutellariae, 4 to 15 g),
30 g • Jie-geng (Radix Platycodi, 2 to 5 g),
30 g • Jing-Jie (Herba Schizonepetae, 5 to
10 g), 15 g • Lian-qiao (Fructus
Forsythiae, 5 to 11 g), 15 g • Ma-huang
(Herba Ephedrae, 5 to 10 g), 15 g •
Mang-xiao (Natrii Sulfas, 4 to 11 g), 15 g
• Shi-gao (Gypsum Fibrosum, 10 to 70 g),
30 g • Zhi-zi (Fructus Gardeniae, 7 to
16 g), 15 g
Instructions: Grind into powder, and
take 9 g of powder twice daily.

52
Formula: *Fang-Ji-Huang-Qi-Tang* (0131)
防已黃芪湯

Ingredients:
Bai-zhu (Rhizoma Atractylodis
Macrocephalae, 5 to 11 g), 10 g • Fang-ji
(Radix Stephaniae Tetrandrae, 5 to 11 g),
15 g • Gan-cao (Radix Glycyrrhizae, 2 to
11 g), 6 g • Huang-qi (Radix Astragali Seu
Hedysari, 5 to 40 g), 30 g

53
Formula: *Feng-Sui-Dan* (0666)
封髓丹

Gan-Cao (Radix Glycyrrhizae, 2 to 11 g),
21 g • Huang-bai (Cortex Phellodendri, 4
to 15 g), 90 g • Sha-ren (Fructus Amomi,
2 to 7 g), 30 g

54
Formula: *Fu-Yuan-Huo-Xue-Tang* (0209)
復元活血湯

Ingredients:
Chai-hu (Radix Bupleuri, 4 to 16 g), 15 g
• Chuan-shan-jia (Squama Manitis, 5 to
11 g), 9 g • Da-huang (Radix Et Rhizoma
Rhei, 4 to 15 g), 30 g • Dang-gui (Radix
Angelicae Sinensis, 5 to 11 g), 9 g • Gan-
cao (Radix Glycyrrhizae, 2 to 11 g), 9 g •
Hong-hua (Flos Carthami, 4 to 7 g), 9 g •
Tao-ren (Semen Persicae, 5 to 11 g), 50
kernels • Tian-hua-fen (Radix
Trichosanthis, 10 to 14 g), 12 g

55
Formula: *Fu-Zi-Li-Zhong-Tang* (0062A)
附子理中湯

Ingredients:
(Use 90 g of each ingredient.)
Bai-zhu (Rhizoma Atractylodis
Macrocephalae, 5 to 11 g) • Fu-zi (Radix
Aconiti Praeparata, 4 to 11 g) • Gan-cao,
zhi-gan-cao (Radix Glycyrrhizae, 2 to 11 g)
• Gan-jiang (Rhizoma Zingiberis, 3 to 7 g)
• Ren-shen (Radix Ginseng, 1 to 35 g)
Instructions: Take 10 g in tablet form
each time; reduce the quantity in
decoction.

56
Formula: *Gan-Mai-Da-Zao-Tang* (0489)
甘麥大枣湯

Ingredients:
Da-zao (Fructus Ziziphi Jujubae, 7 to
18 g), 10 red dates • Gan-cao (Radix
Glycyrrhizae, 2 to 11 g), 9 g • Xiao-mai
(wheat 20 to 50 g), 30 g

57
Formula: *Ge-Gen-Qin-Lian-Tang* (1509)
葛根芩連湯

Ingredients:
Gan-cao (Radix Glycyrrhizae, 2 to 11 g),
60 g • Ge-gen (Radix Puerariae, 4 to
20 g), 240 g • Huang-lian (Rhizoma
Coptidis, 2 to 12 g), 90 g • Huang-qin
(Radix Scutellariae, 4 to 15 g), 90 g

Instructions: Grind into powder, and take 6 g of powder twice daily.

58
Formula: *Ge-Xia-Zhu-Yu-Tang* (0119)

膈下逐瘀湯

Ingredients:

Chi-shao-yao (Radix Paeoniae Rubra, 5 to 11 g), 9 g • *Chuan-xiong* (Rhizoma Ligustici Chuanxiong, 2 to 6 g), 9 g • *Dang-gui* (Radix Angelicae Sinensis, 5 to 11 g), 9 g • *Gan-cao* (Radix Glycyrrhizae, 2 to 11 g), 3 g • *Hong-hua* (Flos Carthami, 4 to 7 g), 6 g • *Mu-dan-pi* (Cortex Moutan Radicis, 5 to 11 g), 6 g • *Tao-ren* (Semen Persicae, 5 to 11 g), 9 g • *Wu-ling-zhi* (Faeces Trogopterorum, 5 to 11 g), 9 g • *Wu-yao* (Radix Linderae, 5 to 10 g), 12 g • *Xiang-fu* (Rhizoma Cyperi, 5 to 11 g), 12 g • *Yan-hu-suo* (Rhizoma Corydalis, 4 to 11 g), 9 g • *Zhi-qiao* (Fructus Aurautii, 4 to 11 g), 9 g

59
Formula: *Gua-Lou-Xie-Bai-Bai-Jiu-Tang* (0215A)

栝楼薤白白酒湯

Ingredients:

Gua-lou (Fructus Trichosanthis, 11 to 15 g), 24 g • *Xie-bai* (Bulbus Allii Macrostemi, 5 to 11 g), 30 g
Instructions: Add wine to decoct in water, or grind into powder and take 6 g of powder with a half glass of wine.

60
Formula: *Gua-Lou-Xie-Bai-Ban-Xia-Tang* (0215B)

栝楼薤白半夏湯

Ingredients:

Ban-xia (Rhizoma Pinelliae, 4 to 12 g), 15 g • *Gua-lou* (Fructus Trichosanthis, 11 to 15 g), 24 g • *Xie-bai* (Bulbus Allii Macrostemi, 5 to 11 g), 20 g

Instructions: Add wine to decoct in water, or grind into powder and take 6 g of powder with a half glass of wine.

61
Formula: *Guan-Xin-Er-Hao-Fang* (0198A)

冠心二號方

Ingredients:

Chi-shao-yao (Radix Paeoniae Rubra, 5 to 11 g), 15 g • *Chuan-xiong* (Rhizoma Ligustici Chuanxiong, 2 to 6 g), 15 g • *Dan-shen* (Radix Salviae Miltiorrhizae, 5 to 10 g), 30 g • *Hong-hua* (Flos Carthami, 4 to 7 g), 15 g • *Jiang-xiang* (Lignum Acronychiae, 15 to 30 g), 10 g

62
Formula: *Gui-Pi-Tang* (0173)

歸脾湯

Ingredients:

Bai-zhu (Rhizoma Atractylodis Macrocephalae, 5 to 11 g), 10 g • *Dang-gui* (Radix Angelicae Sinensis, 5 to 11 g), 12 g • *Dang-shen* (Radix Codonopsis Pilosulae, 11 to 15 g), 12 g • *Fu-shen* (Buyury with pine root, 11 to 15 g), 12 g • *Gan-cao* (Radix Glycyrrhizae, 2 to 11 g), 6 g • *Huang-qi* (Radix Astragali Seu Hedysari, 5 to 40 g), 20 g • *Long-yan-rou* (Arillus Longan, 4 to 11 g), 15 g • *Mu-xiang* (Radix Aucklandiae/Radix Saussureae, 2 to 6 g), 3 g • *Suan-zao-ren* (Semen Ziziphi Spinosae, 7 to 18 g), 15 g • *Yuan-zhi* (Radix Polygalae, 4 to 11 g), 6 g

63
Formula: *Gui-Shao-Di-Huang-Tang* (0996)

歸芍地黃湯

Ingredients:

Bai-shao-yao (Radix Paeoniae Alba, 5 to 11 g), 120 g • *Dang-gui* (Radix Angelicae Sinensis, 5 to 11 g), 120 g • *Fu-ling* (Poria, 7 to 14 g), 90 g • *Mu-dan-pi*

(Cortex Moutan Radicis, 5 to 11 g), 90 g • Shan-yao (Rhizoma Dioscoreae Bulbiferae, 10 to 20 g), 120 g • Shan-zhu-yu (Fructus Corni, 5 to 11 g), 120 g • Sheng-di (Radix Rehmanniae, 14 to 35 g), 240 g • Ze-xie (Rhizoma Alismatis, 7 to 14 g), 90 g

Instructions: Grind into powder to make tablets, and take 9 g of tablets twice daily.

64
Formula: *Gui-Zhi-Fu-Ling-Wan* (0204)

桂枝茯苓丸

Ingredients:
(Use equal quantities of all ingredients.)
Chi-shao-yao (Radix Paeoniae Rubra, 5 to 11 g) • Fu-ling (Poria, 7 to 14 g) • Gui-zhi (Ramulus Cinnamomi, 2 to 10 g) • Mu-dan-pi (Cortex Moutan Radicis, 5 to 11 g) • Tao-ren (Semen Persicae, 5 to 11 g)

Instructions: Grind into powder to make tablets with honey, and take 10 g of tablets each time.

65
Formula: *Gui-Zhi-Gan-Cao-Tang* (0309)

桂枝甘草湯

Ingredients:
Gan-cao (Radix Glycyrrhizae, 2 to 11 g), 6 g • Gui-zhi (Ramulus Cinnamomi, 2 to 10 g), 12 g

66
Formula: *Gui-Zhi-Shao-Yao-Zhi-Mu-Tang* (0003K)

桂枝芍藥知母湯

Ingredients:
Bai-shao-yao (Radix Paeoniae Alba, 5 to 11 g), 10 g • Bai-zhu (Rhizoma Atractylodis Macrocephalae, 5 to 11 g), 15 g • Fang-feng (Radix Ledebouriellae, 5 to 10 g), 10 g • Fu-zi (Radix Aconiti

Praeparata, 4 to 11 g), 6 g • Gan-cao (Radix Glycyrrhizae, 2 to 11 g), 6 g • Gui-zhi (Ramulus Cinnamomi, 2 to 10 g), 10 g • Ma-huang (Herba Ephedrae, 5 to 10 g), 6 g • Sheng-jiang (Rhizoma Zingiberis Recens, 4 to 10 g), 10 g • Zhi-mu (Rhizoma Anemarrhenae, 4 to 15 g), 10 g

67
Formula: *He-Che-Wan* (1153)

河車丸

Ingredients:
Dan-shen (Radix Salviae Miltiorrhizae, 5 to 10 g), 18 g • Fu-ling (Poria, 7 to 14 g), 30 g • Fu-shen (Buyury with pine root, 11 to 15 g), 30 g • Ren-shen (Radix Ginseng, 1 to 35 g), 15 g • Yuan-zhi (Radix Polygalae, 4 to 11 g), 30 g • Zi-he-che (Placenta Hominis, 2 to 5 g), 25 g

Instructions: Grind into powder to make tablets, and take 9 g of tablets twice daily.

68
Formula: *Hou-Pu-San-Wu-Tang* (0670)

厚朴三物湯

Ingredients:
Da-huang (Radix Et Rhizoma Rhei, 4 to 15 g), 15 g • Hou-po (Cortex Magnoliae Officinalis, 4 to 11 g), 18 g • Zhi-shi (Fructus Aurantii Immaturus, 4 to 7 g), 15 g

69
Formula: *Huai-Hua-San* (0223)

槐花散

Ingredients:
Ce-bai-ye (Caumen Biotae, 7 to 14 g), 15 g • Huai-hua (Flos Sophorae, 5 to 11 g), 30 g • Jing-jie (Herba Schizonepetae, 5 to 10 g), 9 g • Zhi-qiao (Fructus Aurantii, 4 to 11 g), 9 g

70

Formula: *Huang-Lian-E-Jiao-Tang* (0302)

黃連阿膠湯

Ingredients:

Bai-shao yao (Radix Paeoniae Alba, 5 to 11 g), 15 g • E-jiao (Colla Corii Asini, 5 to 11 g), 12 g • Huang-lian (Rhizoma Coptidis, 2 to 12 g), 6 g • Huang-qin (Radix Scutellariae, 4 to 15 g), 12 g • Ji-zi-huang (Chicken egg yolk, 10 to 20 g), one egg

71

Formula: *Huang-Lian-Tang* (0105e)

黃連湯

Ingredients:

Ban-xia (Rhizoma Pinelliae, 4 to 12 g), 15 g • Da-zao (Fructus Ziziphi Jujubae, 7 to 18 g), 9 g • Gan-cao, Zhi-Gan-Cao (Radix Glycyrrhizae, 2 to 11 g), 3 g • Gan-jiang (Rhizoma Zingiberis, 3 to 7 g), 9 g • Gui-zhi (Ramulus Cinnamomi, 2 to 10 g), 9 g • Huang-lian (Rhizoma Coptidis, 2 to 12 g), 6 g • Ren-shen (Radix Ginseng, 1 to 35 g), 9 g

72

Formula: *Huang-Qin-Qing-Fei-Yin* (0786)

黃芩清肺飲

Ingredients:

Huang-qin (Radix Scutellariae, 4 to 15 g), 3 g • Zhi-zi (Fructus Gardeniae, 7 to 16 g), 3 g

73

Formula: *Huang-Tu-Tang* (0144)

黃土湯

Ingredients:

Bai-zhu (Rhizoma Atractylodis Macrocephalae, 5 to 11 g), 10 g • E-jiao (Colla Corii Asini, 5 to 11 g), 12 g • Fu-long-gan (Terra Flava Usta, 17 to 35 g),
30 g • Fu-zi (Radix Aconiti Praeparata, 4 to 11 g), 10 g • Gan-cao (Radix Glycyrrhizae, 2 to 11 g), 3 g • Gan-di dried Radix Rehmanniae, 11 to 18 g), 15 g • Huang-qin (Radix Scutellariae, 4 to 15 g), 12 g

74

Formula: *Huo-Pu-Xia-Ling-Tang* (0118)

藿朴夏苓湯

Ingredients:

Bai-dou-kou (Fructus Amomi Cardamomi, 2 to 7 g), 3 g • Ban-xia (Rhizoma Pinelliae, 4 to 12 g), 10 g • Dan-dou-chi (Semen Sojae Praeparatum, 7 to 14 g), 10 g • Fu-ling (Poria, 7 to 14 g), 10 g • Hou-po (Cortex Magnoliae Officinalis, 4 to 11 g), 6 g • Huo-xiang (Herba Agastachis, 5 to 11 g), 10 g • Xing-ren (Semen Armeniacae Amarae, 5 to 11 g), 6 g • Yi-yi-ren (Semen Coicis, 11 to 22 g), 20 g • Ze-xie (Rhizoma Alismatis, 7 to 14 g), 6 g • Zhu-ling (Polyporus Umbellatus, 7 to 14 g), 6 g

75

Formula: *Huo-Xiang-Zheng-Qi-San* (0101)

藿香正氣散

Ingredients:

Bai-zhi (Radix Angelicae Dahuricae, 4 to 10 g), 9 g • Bai-zhu (Rhizoma Atractylodis Macrocephalae, 5 to 11 g), 9 g • Ban-xia (Rhizoma Pinelliae, 4 to 12 g), 12 g • Chen-pi (Pericarpium Papaveris, 4 to 11 g), 9 g • Da-fu-pi (Pericarpium Papaveris/Fructus Papaveris Arecae, 5 to 18 g), 15 g • Fu-ling (Poria, 7 to 14 g), 12 g • Gan-cao (Radix Glycyrrhizae, 2 to 11 g), 3 g • Hou-po (Cortex Magnoliae Officinalis, 4 to 11 g), 12 g • Huo-xiang (Herba Agastachis, 5 to 11 g), 9 g • Jie-geng (Radix Platycodi, 2 to 5 g), 6 g • Zi-su-ye (Folium Perillae, 5 to 10 g), 9 g

76

Formula: *Ji-Chuan-Jian* (1203)

濟川煎

Ingredients:

Dang-gui (Radix Angelicae Sinensis, 5 to 11 g), 10 g • *Niu-xi (Radix Achyranthis bidentatae* 5 to 11 g), 6 g • *Rou-cong-rong (Herba Cistanchis,* 7 to 11 g), 9 g • *Sheng-ma (Rhizoma Cimicifugae,* 3 to 10 g), 2 g • *Ze-xie (Rhizoma Alismatis,* 7 to 14 g), 4 g • *Zhi-qiao (Fructus Aurantii,* 4 to 11 g), 3 g

77
Formula: *Ji-Sheng-Shen-Qi-Wan* (0331A)

濟生腎氣丸

Ingredients:

Che-qian-zi (Semen Plantaginis, 4 to 11 g), 80 g • *Fu-ling (Poria,* 7 to 14 g), 90 g • *Fu-zi (Radix Aconiti Praeparata,* 4 to 11 g), 30 g • *Gan-di* (dried *Radix Rehmanniae,* 11 to 18 g), 240 g • *Gui-zhi (Ramulus Cinnamomi,* 2 to 10 g), 30 g • *Mu-dan-pi (Cortex Moutan Radicis,* 5 to 11 g), 90 g • *Niu-xi (Radix Achyranthis Bidentatae,* 5 to 11 g), 80 g • *Shan-yao (Rhizoma Dioscoreae,* 10 to 20 g), 120 g • *Shan-zhu-yu (Fructus Corni,* 5 to 11 g), 120 g • *Ze-xie (Rhizoma Alismatis,* 7 to 14 g), 90 g

Instructions: Grind into powder to make tablets with honey. Take 9 g of tablets one to two times daily, with warm or lightly salted water. Use reduced quantities of ingredients if decoction is done.

78
Formula: *Jia-Wei-Er-Chen-Tang* (0121M)

加味二陳湯

Ingredients:

Bai-guo (Semen Ginkgo, 5 to 11 g), 9 g • *Ban-xia (Rhizoma Pinelliae,* 4 to 12 g), 15 g • *Che-qian-zi (Semen Plantaginis,* 4 to 11 g), 9 g • *Chen-pi (Pericarpium Citri Reticulatae,* 4 to 11 g), 10 g • *Chun-bai-pi (Cortex Toona,* 7 to 14 g), 9 g • *Fu-ling (Poria,* 7 to 14 g), 15 g • *Gan-cao (Radix Glycyrrhizae,* 2 to 11 g), 3 g • *Huang-bai (Cortex Phellodendri,* 4 to 15 g), 9 g • *Tian-nan-xing (Rhizoma Arisaematis,* 2.5 to 5 g), 9 g

79
Formula: *Jia-Wei-Shi-Xiao-San* (0201A)

加味失笑散

Ingredients:

(Use equal amounts of all ingredients.)
Mu-dan-pi (Cortex Moutan Radicis, 5 to 11 g) • *Pu-huang (Pollen Typhae,* 5 to 11 g) • *Tao-ren (Semen Persicae,* 5 to 11 g) • *Wu-ling-zhi (Faeces Trogopterorum,* 5 to 11 g) • *Wu-yao (Radix Linderae,* 5 to 10 g) • *Xiang-fu (Rhizoma Cyperi,* 5 to 11 g) • *Xuan-ming-Fen (Mirabilitum Dehydratum,* 4 to 11 g)

Instructions: Grind into powder, and take 9 g of powder two times daily.

80
Formula: *Jia-Wei-Si-Ling-San* (0348F)

加味四苓散

Ingredients:

Bai-zhu (Rhizoma Atractylodis Macrocephalae, 5 to 11 g), 9 g • *Chen-pi (Pericarpium Papaveris,* 4 to 11 g), 9 g • *Fu-ling (Poria,* 7 to 14 g), 12 g • *Hou-po (Cortex Magnoliae Officinalis,* 4 to 11 g), 12 g • *Ze-xie (Rhizoma Alismatis,* 7 to 14 g), 15 g • *Zhu-ling (Polyporus Umbellatus,* 7 to 14 g), 12 g

81
Formula: *Jian-Ling-Tang* (0242B)

建瓴湯

Ingredients:

Bai-shao-yao (Radix Paeoniae Alba, 5 to 11 g), 12 g • *Bai-zi-ren (Semen Biotae,* 4 to 11 g), 12 g • *Dai-zhe-shi (Ocherum Rubrum,* 1 to 35 g), 24 g • *Long-gu (Os Draconis,* 11 to 18 g), 18 g • *Mu-li (Concha Ostrae,* 11 to 35 g), 18 g • *Niu-xi (Radix Achyranthis Bidentatae,* 5 to

11 g), 30 g • *Shan-yao (Rhizoma Dioscoreae,* 10 to 20 g), 30 g • *Sheng-di (Radix Rehmanniae,* 14 to 35 g), 18 g

82
Formula: *Jiang-Tang-Er-Hao-Fang* (3362)

降糖二號方

Ingredients:

Bai-zhu (Rhizoma Atractylodis Macrocephalae, 5 to 11 g), 30 g • *He-shou-Wu (Radix Polygoni Multiflori,* 11 to 15 g), 30 g • *Huang-qi (Radix Astragali Seu Hedysari,* 5 to 40 g), 30 g • *Shan-yao (Rhizoma Dioscoreae,* 10 to 20 g), 30 g • *Sheng-di (Radix Rehmanniae,* 14 to 35 g), 24 g • *Shi-gao (Gypsum Fibrosum,* 10 to 70 g), 30 g • *Shu-di-huang (Radix Rehmanniae Praeparatae,* 11 to 18 g), 30 g • *Tian-dong (Radix Asparagi,* 7 to 14 g), 15 g • *Tian-hua-Fen (Radix Trichosanthis,* 10 to 14 g), 90 g • *Xuan-shen (Radix Scrophulariae,* 7 to 35 g), 24 g • *Yu-zhu (Rhizoma Polygonati Odorati,* 5 to 11 g), 20 g • *Zhi-mu (Rhizoma Anemarrhenae,* 4 to 15 g), 15 g

83
Formula: *Jiang-Tang-San-Hao-Fang* (3363)

降糖三號方

Ingredients:

Bai-zhu (Rhizoma Atractylodis Macrocephalae 5 to 11 g), 30 g • *Gou-qi-zi (Fructus Lych,* 5 to 11 g), 30 g • *He-shou-wu (Radix Polygoni Multiflori,* 11 to 15 g), 30 g • *Huang-bai (Cortex Phellodendri,* 4 to 15 g), 12 g • *Huang-qi (Radix Astragali Seu Hedysari,* 5 to 40 g), 30 g • *Sang-piao-xiao (Ootheca Mantidis,* 5 to 11 g), 12 g • *Shan-yao (Rhizoma Dioscoreae,* 10 to 20 g), 40 g • *Shan-zhu-yu (Fructus Corni,* 5 to 11 g), 18 g • *Sheng-di (Radix Rehmanniae,* 14 to 35 g), 20 g • *Shu-di-huang (Radix Rehmanniae Praeparatae,* 11 to 18 g), 20 g • *Tian-hua-fen (RAdix Trichosanthis,* 10 to 14 g), 12 g • *Xuan-shen (Radix Scrophulariae,* 7 to 35 g), 20 g

84
Formula: *Jiang-Tang-Si-Hao-Fang* (3364)

降糖四號方

Ingredients:

Bai-zhu (Rhizoma Atractylodis Macrocephalae, 5 to 11 g), 30 g • *Cang-zhu (Rhizoma Atractylodis,* 4 to 11 g), 15 g • *Ge-gen (Radix Puerariae,* 4 to 20 g), 12 g • *Gou-qi-zi (Fructus Lych,* 5 to 11 g), 30 g • *He-shou-wu (Radix Polygoni Multiflori,* 11 to 15 g), 30 g • *Huang-jing (Rhizoma Polygonati,* 11 to 15 g), 30 g • *Huang-qi (Radix Astragali Seu Hedysari,* 5 to 40 g), 20 g • *Shan-yao (Rhizoma Dioscoreae,* 10 to 20 g), 30 g • *Sheng-di (Radix Rehmanniae,* 14 to 35 g), 20 g • *Tian-hua-fen (Radix Trichosanthis,* 10 to 14 g), 30 g • *Xuan-Shen (Radix Scrophulariae,* 7 to 35 g), 30 g

85
Formula: *Jiang-Tang-Yi-Hao-Fang* (3361)

降糖一號方

Ingredients:

Bei-sha-shen (Radix Glehniae, 5 to 11 g), 24 g • *Shan-yao (Rhizoma Dioscoreae,* 10 to 20 g), 45 g • *Sheng-di (Radix Rehmanniae,* 14 to 35 g), 30 g • *Shi-gao (Gypsum Fibrosum,* 10 to 70 g), 60 g • *Tian-Dong (Radix Asparagi,* 7 to 14 g), 20 g • *Tian-hua-fen (Radix Trichosanthis,* 10 to 14 g), 120 g • *Xuan-shen (Radix Scrophulariae,* 7 to 35 g), 30 g • *Yu-zhu (Rhizoma Polygonati Odorati,* 5 to 11 g), 20 g • *Zhi-mu (Rhizoma Anemarrhenae,* 4 to 15 g), 18 g

86
Formula: *Jin-Suo-Gu-Jing-Wan* (0342)

金鎖固精丸

Ingredients:

Lian-xu (Stamen Nelumbinis, 3 to 7 g), 60 g • *Long-gu, duan-long-gu (OS Draconis,* 11 to 18 g), 30 g • *Mu-li duan-*

mu-li (Concha Ostrae, 11 to 35 g), 30 g •
Qian-shi (Semen Euryales, 7 to 11 g), 60 g
• Sha-wan-zi (Semen Astragalus, 7 to
11 g), 60 g

Instructions: Grind into powder to make
tablets with cooked lotus powder, and
take 9 g of tablets twice daily.

87
Formula: Jing-Fang-Bai-Du-San (0004B)

荊防敗毒散

Ingredients:
Chai-hu (Radix Bupleuri, 4 to 16 g), 10 g
• Chuan-xiong (Rhizoma Ligustici
Chuanxiong, 2 to 6 g), 10 g • Du-huo
(Radix Angelicae Pubescentis, 2 to 5 g),
10 g • Fang-feng (Radix Ledebouriellae, 5
to 10 g), 10 g • Fu-ling (Poria, 7 to
14 g), 10 g • Gan-cao (Radix
Glycyrrhizae, 2 to 11 g), 3 g • Jing-jie
(Herba Schizonepetae, 5 to 10 g), 10 g •
Jie-geng (Radix Platycodi, 2 to 5 g), 10 g •
Qian-hu Radix Peucedani, 5 to 11 g), 10 g
• Qiang-huo (Rhizoma Seu Radix
Notopterygii, 4 to 10 g), 10 g • Zhi-qiao
(Fructus Auranth, 4 to 11 g), 10 g

88
Formula: Ju-Fang-Zhi-Bao-Dan (1823)

局方至寶丹

Ingredients:
An-xi-xiang (Benzoinum, 0.3 to 2 g), 45 g
• Bing-pian (Borneol, 0.2 to 0.3 g), 7.5 g •
Dai-mao (Carapax Eretmochelydis
Erethmochelyos, 4 to 7 g), 30 g • Hu-po
(Succinum, 1 to 2 g), 30 g • Jin-bo
(Native Gold Slice flexible g,) 50 g • Niu-
huang (Calculus Bovis, 0.2 to 0.5 g), 15 g
• She-xiang (Moschus, 0.01 to 0.03 g),
7.5 g • Xi-jiao (Cornu Rhinoceri, 1 to
2 g), 30 g • Xiong-huang (Realgar, 03. to
1.5 g), 30 g • Yin-bo (Native Silver Slice
flexible g), 50 g • Zhu-sha (Cinnabaris,
0.3 to 1 g), 30 g

Instructions: Grind into powder to make
tablets, and take 3 g of tablets twice
daily.

89
Formula: Juan-Bi-Tang (1485)

蠲痺湯

Ingredients:
Chuan-xiong (Rhizoma Ligustici
Chuanxiong 2 to 6 g), 2 g • Dang-gui
(Radix Angelicae Sinensis, 5 to 11 g), 9 g •
Du-huo (Radix Angelicae Pubescentis, 2 to
5 g), 3 g • Gan-cao (Radix Glycyrrhizae, 2
to 11 g), 1.5 g • Hai-feng-teng (Caulis
Piperis Futokadsurae, 7 to 18 g), 6 g •
Jiang-huang (Rhizoma Curcumae Longae, 4
to 11 g), 6 g • Mu-xiang (Radix
Aucklandiae/Radix Saussureae, 2 to 6 g),
2 g • Qiang-huo (Rhizoma Seu Radix
Notopterygii, 4 to 10 g), 3 g • Qin-jiao
(Radix Gentianae Macrophyllae, 4 to 11 g),
3 g • Rou-gui (Cortex Cinnamomi, 1 to
5 g), 1.5 g • Ru-xiang (Mastix/resina, 4
to 11 g), 2 g • Sang-zhi (Ramulus Mori,
11 to 18 g), 9 g

90
Formula: Kai-Guan-San (0438)

開關散

Ingredients:
Bai-zhi (Radix Angelicae Dahuricae, 4 to
10 g), 2 g • Chuan-xiong (Rhizoma
Ligustici Chuanxiong, 2 to 6 g), 3 g

Instructions: Grind into powder for
consumption as one dose, and take two
doses daily.

91
Formula: Ke-Xue-Tang (0280)

咳血方

Ingredients:
Gua-lou-ren (Semen Trichosanthis, 11 to
15 g), 9 g • Hai-fu-shi (Pumex, 10 to
18 g), 9 g • He-zi (Fructus Chebulae, 2 to
5 g), 9 g • Qing-dai (Indigo Naturalis, 2
to 4 g), 9 g • Zhi-zi (Fructus Gardeniae, 7
to 16 g), 9 g

92
Formula: *Li-Zhong-Wan* (0062)

理中丸

Ingredients:
(Use 90 g of each ingredient.)
Bai-zhu (Rhizoma Atractylodis Macrocephalae, 5 to 11 g) • *Gan-cao, zhi-gan-cao (Radix Glycyrrhizae, 2 to 11 g)* • *Gan-jiang (Rhizoma Zingiberis, 3 to 7 g)* • *Ren-shen (Radix Ginseng, 1 to 35 g)*
Instructions: Take 10 g in tablet form each time; reduce the quantity if decoction is done.

93
Formula: *Ling-Gui-Zhu-Gan-Tang* (0119)

苓桂术甘湯

Ingredients:
Bai-zhu (Rhizoma Atractylodis Macrocephalae, 5 to 11 g), 15 g • *Fu-ling (Poria, 7 to 14 g)*, 20 g • *Gan-cao (Radix Glycyrrhizae, 2 to 11 g)*, 6 g • *Gui-zhi (Ramulus Cinnamomi, 2 to 10 g)*, 15 g

94
Formula: *Ling-Yang-Gou-Teng-Tang* (0243)

羚角钩藤湯

Ingredients:
Bai-shao-yao (Radix Paeoniae Alba, 5 to 11 g), 30 to 60 g • *Chuan-bei-mu (Bulbus Fritillariae Cirrhosae, 4 to 14 g)*, 6 g • *Fu-shen (Buyury with pine root, 11 to 15 g)*, 15 g • *Gan-cao (Radix Glycyrrhizae, 2 to 11 g)*, 6 g • *Gou-teng (Ramulus Uncariae Cum Uncis, 5 to 11 g)*, 12 g • *Ju-hua (Flos Chrysanthemi, 4 to 20 g)*, 12 g • *Ling-yang-Jiao (Cornu Antelopis, 1 to 1.5 g)*, 9 g • *Sang-ye (Folium Mori, 5 to 10 g)*, 9 g • *Sheng-di (Radix Rehmanniae, 14 to 35 g)*, 24 g • *Zhu-ru (Caulis Bambusae in Taeniam, 5 to 11 g)*, 12 g

95
Formula: *Liu-Jun-Zi-Tang* (0080C)

六君子湯

Ingredients:
Bai-zhu (Rhizoma Atractylodis Macrocephalae, 5 to 11 g), 10 g • *Ban-xia (Rhizoma Pinelliae, 4 to 12 g)*, 10 g • *Cheng-pi (Pericarpium Papaveris, 4 to 11 g)*, 10 g • *Fu-ling (Poria, 7 to 14 g)*, 12 g • *Gan-cao (Radix Clycyrrhizae, 2 to 11 g)*, 3 g • *Ren-shen (Radix Ginseng, 1 to 35 g)*, 15 g

96
Formula: *Liu-Mo-Yin* (0419)

六磨飲

Ingredients:
Bing-lang (Semen Areca, 4 to 11 g), 6 g • *Chen-xiang (Lignum Aquilariae Resinatum, 1 to 4 g)*, 3 g • *Da-huang (Radix Et Rhizoma Rhei, 4 to 15 g)*, 8 g • *Mu-xiang (Radix Aucklandiae/Radix Saussureae, 2 to 6 g)*, 4 g • *Wu-yao (Radix Linderae, 5 to 10 g)*, 7 g • *Zhi-shi (Fructus Aurantii Immaturus, 4 to 7 g)*, 5 g

97
Formula: *Liu-Wei-Di-Huang-Wan* (0307)

六味地黃丸

Ingredients:
Fu-ling (Poria, 7 to 14 g), 90 g • *Mu-dan-pi (Cortex Moutan Radicis, 5 to 11 g)*, 90 g • *Shan-yao (Rhizoma Dioscoreae, 10 to 20 g)*, 120 g • *Shan-zhu-yu (Fructus Corni, 5 to 11 g)*, 120 g • *Shu-di-huang (Radix Rehmanniae Praeparatae, 11 to 18 g)*, 240 g • *Ze-xie (Rhizoma Alismatis, 7 to 14 g)*, 90 g
Instructions: Grind into powder to make tablets, and take three tablets or 9 g two to three times daily.

98
Formula: *Long-Dan-Xie-Gan-Tang* (0188)

龍膽瀉肝湯

Ingredients:
Chai-hu (Radix Bupleuri, 4 to 16 g), 9 g • Che-qian-zi (Semen Plantaginis, 4 to 11 g), 12 g • Dang-gui (Radix Angelicae Sinensis, 5 to 11 g), 9 g • Gan-cao (Radix Glycyrrhizae, 2 to 11 g), 3 g • Huang-qin (Radix Scutellariae, 4 to 15 g), 12 g • Long-dan (Radix Gentianae, 7 to 10 g), 9 g • Mu-tong (Caulis Aristologhiae, 4 to 8 g), 12 g • Sheng-di (Radix Rehmanniae, 14 to 35 g), 15 g • Ze-xie (Rhizoma Alismatis, 7 to 14 g), 9 g • Zhi-zi (Fructus Gardeniae, 7 to 16 g), 9 g

99
Formula: *Ma-Huang-Lian-Qiao-Chi-Xiao-Dou-Tang* (0059)

麻黃連翹赤小豆湯

Ingredients:
Chi-xiao-dou (Semen Phaseoli, 11 to 18 g), 15 g • Da-zao (Fructus Ziziphi Jujubae, 7 to 18 g), 4 dates • Gan-cao (Radix Glycyrrhizae, 2 to 11 g), 6 g • Lian-qiao (Fructus Forsythiae, 5 to 11 g), 15 g • Ma-huang (Herba Ephedrae, 5 to 10 g), 9 g • Sheng-jiang (Rhizoma Zingiberis Recens, 4 to 10 g), 9 g • Xing-ren (Semen Armeniacae Amarae, 5 to 11 g), 9 g • Zi-bai-pi (Cortex Catalpa 5 to 15 g), 15 g

100
Formula: *Ma-Xing-Shi-Gan-Tang* (0028)

麻杏石甘湯

Ingredients:
Gan-cao (Radix Glycyrrhizae, 2 to 11 g), 3 g • Ma-huang (Herba Ephedrae, 5 to 10 g), 9 g • Shi-gao (Gypsum Fibrosum, 10 to 70 g), 30 g • Xing-ren (Semen Armeniacae Amarae, 5 to 11 g), 9 g.

101
Formula: *Ma-Zi-Ren-Wan* (0161)

麻子仁湯

Ingredients:
Chi-shao-yao (Radix Paeoniae Rubra, 5 to 11 g), 15 g • Da-Huang (Radix Et

Rhizoma Rhei, 4 to 15 g), 20 g • Hou-po (Cortex Magnoliae Officinalis, 4 to 11 g), 15 g • Huo-ma-ren (Fructus Cannabis, 11 to 17 g), 30 g • Xing-ren (Semen Armeniacae Amarae, 5 to 11 g), 15 g • Zhi-shi (Fructus Aurantii Immaturus, 4 to 7 g), 10 g

102
Formula: *Mai-Men-Dong-Tang* (0140)

麥門冬湯

Ingredients:
Ban-xia (Rhizoma Pinelliae, 4 to 12 g), 10 g • Da-zao (Fructus Ziziphi Jujubae, 7 to 18 g), 10 g • Gan-cao (Radix Glycyrrhizae, 2 to 11 g), 6 g • Jing-Mi (Polished rice, flexible quantity), 10 g • Mai-men-dong (Radix Ophiopogonis, 5 to 11 g), 30 g • Ren-shen (Radix Ginseng, 1 to 35 g), 6g

103
Formula: *Mai-Wei-Di-Huang-Wan* (0327C)

麥味地黃丸

Ingredients:
Fu-ling (Poria, 7 to 14 g), 90 g • Mai-men-dong (Radix Ophiopogonis, 5 to 11 g), 90 g • Mu-dan-pi (Cortex Moutan Radicis, 5 to 11 g), 90 g • Shan-yao (Rhizoma Dioscoreae, 10 to 20 g), 120 g • Shan-zhu-yu (Fructus Corni, 5 to 11 g), 120 g • Shu-di-huang (Radix Rehmanniae Praeparatae, 11 to 18 g), 240 g • Wu-wei-zi (Fructus Schisandrae, 2 to 4 g), 90 g • Ze-xie (Rhizoma Alismatis, 7 to 14 g), 90 g
Instructions: Grind into powder to make tablets, and take three tablets or 9 g two to three times daily.

104
Formula: *Mi-Niao-Xi-Tong-Gan-Ran-He-Ji* (1903)

泌尿系感梁合劑

Ingredients:
Chai-hu (Radix Bupleuri, 4 to 16 g), 25 g • Che-qian-Zi (Semen Plantaginis, 4 to

11 g), 15 g • Huang-bai (Cortex Phellodendri, 4 to 15 g), 15 g • Huang-qin (Radix Scutellariae, 4 to 15 g), 15 g • Wu-wei-zi (Fructus Schisandrae, 2 to 4 g), 15 g

105

Formula: Mu-Xiang-Bing-Lang-Wan (0076)

木香檳榔丸

Ingredients:

Bing-lang (Semen Areca, 4 to 11 g), 15 g • Chen-pi (Pericarpium Papaveris, 4 to 11 g), 15 g • Da-huang (Radix Et Rhizoma Rhei, 4 to 15 g), 30 g • E-zhu (Rhizoma Zedoariae, 5 to 11 g), 15 g • Huang-bai (Cortex Phellodendri, 4 to 15 g), 15 g • Huang-lian (Rhizoma Coptidis, 2 to 12 g), 15 g • Mu-xiang (Radix Aucklandiae/Radix Saussureae, 2 to 6 g), 15 g • Qian-niu-zi (Semen Pharbitidis, 4 to 7 g), 60 g • Qing-pi (Pericarpium Papaveris, 4 to 11 g), 15 g • Xiang-fu (Rhizoma Cyperi, 5 to 11 g), 60 g

106

Formula: Mu-Xiang-Shun-Qi-Wan (0442)

木香順氣丸

Ingredients:

Bing-lang (Semen Areca, 4 to 11 g), 30 g • Cang-zhu (Rhizoma Atractylodis Macrocephalae, 4 to 11 g), 30 g • Chen-pi (Pericarpium Citri Reticulatae Viride, 4 to 11 g), 30 g • Gan-cao (Radix Glycyrrhizae, 2 to 11 g), 15 g • Hou-po (Cortex Magnoliae Officinalis, 4 to 11 g), 30 g • Mu-xiang (Radix Aucklandiae/Radix Saussureae, 2 to 6 g), 30 g • Qing-pi (Pericarpium Citri Reticulatae Viride, 4 to 11 g), 30 g • Sha-ren (Fructus Amomi, 2 to 7 g), 30 g • Xiang-fu (Rhizoma Cyperi, 5 to 11 g), 30 g • Zhi-Qiao (Fructus Aurantii, 4 to 11 g), 30 g

Instructions: Grind into powder, and take 9 g of powder twice daily.

107

Formula: Ping-Wei-San (0117)

平胃散

Ingredients:

Cang-zhu (Rhizoma Atractylodis Macrocephalae, 4 to 11 g), 10 g • Chen-pi (Pericarpium Papaveris, 4 to 11 g), 10 g • Gan-cao (Radix Glycyrrhizae, 2 to 11 g), 3 g • Hou-po (Cortex Magnoliae Officinalis, 4 to 11 g), 10 g

108

Formula: Qi-Gong-Wan (0559)

啟宮丸

Ingredients:

Ban-xia (Rhizoma Pinelliae, 4 to 12 g), 45 g • Cang-zhu (Rhizoma Atractylodis Macrocephalae, 4 to 11 g), 60 g • Chen-pi (Pericarpium Citri Reticulatae Viride, 4 to 11 g), 45 g • Chuan-xiong (Rhizoma Ligustici Chuanxiong, 2 to 6 g), 45 g • Fu-ling (Poria, 7 to 14 g) 45 g • Shen-qu (Massa Medicata Fermentata, 7 to 15 g), 45 g • Xiang-fu (Rhizoma Cyperi, 5 to 11 g), 60 g

109

Formula: Qian-Jin-Xi-Jiao-Tang (0411)

千金犀角湯

Ingredients:

Da-huang (Radix Et Rhizoma Rhei, 4 to 15 g), 5 g • Dou-chi (Semen sojae Praeparatum, 10 to 15 g), 8 g • Huang-qin (Radix Scutellariae, 4 to 15 g), 5 g • Ling-yang-Jiao (Cornu Antelopis, 1 to 1.5 g), 1 g • Qian-Hu (Radix Peucedani, 3 to 11 g), 5 g • She-gan (Rhizoma Belamcandae, 2 to 5 g), 3 g • Sheng-ma (Rhizoma Cimicifugae, 3 to 10 g), 6 g • Xi-jiao (Cornu Rhinoceri, 1 to 2 g), 1 g • Zhi-Zi (Fructus Gardeniae, 7 to 16 g), 8 g

110

Formula: Qian-Zheng-San (0253)

牽正散

Ingredients:
(Use equal quantities of all ingredients.)
Du-jiao-lian (Rhizoma Typhonii, external uses) • *Jiang-can (Bombyx Batryticatus, 5 to 11 g)* • *Quan-xie (Scorpio, 2 to 5 g)*

Instructions: Grind into powder, and take 3 g of powder each time with hot wine.

111

Formula: *Qiang-Huo-Sheng-Shi-Tang* (0010)

羌活勝濕湯

Ingredients:
Chuan-xiong (Rhizoma Ligustici Chuanxiong, 2 to 6 g), 6 g • *Du-huo (Radix Angelicae Pubescentis, 2 to 5 g), 9 g* • *Gan-cao (Radix Glycyrrhizae, 2 to 11 g), 3 g* • *Gao-ben (Rhizoma Et Radix Ligustici, 4 to 10 g), 6 g* • *Man-jing-Zi (Fructus Viticis, 4 to 15 g), 6 g* • *Qiang-huo (Rhizoma Seu Radix Notopterygii Notopterygii, 4 to 10 g), 9 g*

112

Formula: *Qin-Jiao-Bie-Jia-San* (0275)

秦艽鱉甲散

Ingredients:
Bie-jia (Carapax Trionycis, 11 to 18 g), 30 g • *Chai-hu (Radix Bupleuri, 4 to 16 g), 30 g* • *Dang-gui (Radix Angelicae Sinensis, 5 to 11 g), 15 g* • *Di-gu-pi (Cortex Lych Radicis, 5 to 11 g), 30 g* • *Qin-jiao (Radix Gentianae Macrophyllae, 4 to 11 g), 15 g* • *Zhi-mu (Rhizoma Anemarrhenae, 4 to 15 g), 15 g*

113

Formula: *Qing-Gan-Tang* (0756)

清肝湯

Ingredients:
Bai-shao-yao (Radix Paeoniae Alba, 5 to 11 g), 5 g • *Chai-hu (Radix Bapleuri, 4 to 16 g), 2 g* • *Chuan-xiong (Rhizoma*

Ligustici Chuanxiong, 2 to 6 g), 3 g • *Dang-gui (Radix Angelicae Sinensis, 5 to 11 g), 3 g* • *Mu-dan-pi (Cortex Moutan Radicis, 5 to 11 g), 1.5 g* • *Zhi-zi (Fructus Gardeniae, 7 to 16 g), 1.5 g*

114

Formula: *Qing-Gong-Tang* (0281A)

清宮湯

Ingredients:
Lian-Qiao (Fructus Forsythiae, 5 to 11 g), 6 g • *Lian-zi-xin (Plumula Nelumbinis, 2 to 4 g), 3 g* • *Mai-men-dong (Radix Ophiopogonis, 5 to 11 g), 9 g* • *Xi-jiao (Cornu Rhinoceri, 1 to 2 g), 2 to 3 g* • *Xuan-shen (Radix Scrophulariae, 7 to 35 g), 12 g* • *Zhu-juan-xin (young bamboo leaf, 3 to 5 g), 6 g*

115

Formula: *Qing-Gu-Zi-Shen-Tang* (0755)

清骨滋腎湯

Ingredients:
Bai-zhu (Rhizoma Atractylodis Macrocephalae, 5 to 11 g), 10 g • *Bei-sha-shen (Radix Glehniae, 5 to 11 g), 15 g* • *Di-gu-pi (Cortex Lych Radicis, 5 to 11 g), 30 g* • *Mai-men-dong (Radix Ophiopogonis, 5 to 11 g), 15 g* • *Mu-dan-pi (Cortex Moutan Radicis, 5 to 11 g), 15 g* • *Shi-hu (Herba Dendrobii, 7 to 14 g), 6 g* • *Wu-wei-zi (Fructus Schisandrae, 2 to 4 g), 1.5 g* • *Xuan-shen (Radix Scrophulariae, 7 to 35 g), 15 g*

116

Formula: *Qing-Hao-Bie-Jia-Tang* (0277)

青蒿鱉甲湯

Ingredients:
Bie-jia (Carapax Trionycis, 11 to 18 g), 15 g • *Mu-dan-pi (Cortex Moutan Radicis, 5 to 11 g), 9 g* • *Qing-hao (Herba Artemisiae Chinghao, 5 to 11 g), 15 g* • *Sheng-di (Radix Rehmanniae, 14 to 35 g),*

12 g • Zhi-mu (Rhizoma Anemarrhenae, 4 to 15 g), 9 g

117
Formula: Qing-Jing-Tang (0272A)

清經湯

Ingredients:

Bai-shao-yao (Radix Paeoniae Alba, 5 to 11 g), 12 g • Di-gu-pi (Cortex Lych Radicis, 5 to 11 g), 12 g • Fu-ling (Poria, 7 to 14 g), 9 g • Huang-bai (Cortex Phellodendri, 4 to 15 g), 9 g • Mu-dan-pi (Cortex Moutan Radicis, 5 to 11 g), 9 g • Qing-hao (Herba Artemisiae Chinghao, 5 to 11 g), 12 g • Shu-di-huang (Radix Rehmanniae Praeparatae, 11 to 18 g), 15 g

118
Formula: Qing-Xue-Yang-Yin-Tang (0754)

清血養陰湯

Ingredients:

Bai-shao-yao (Radix Paeoniae Alba, 5 to 11 g), 8 g • Huang-bai (Cortex Phellodendri, 4 to 15 g), 9 g • Mo-han-lian (Herba Ecliptae, 5 to 11 g), 7 g • Mu-dan-pi (Cortex Moutan Radicis, 5 to 11 g), 8 g • Nu-zhen-zi (Fructus Ligustri Lucidi, 5 to 11 g), 7 g • Sheng-di (Radix Rehmanniae, 14 to 35 g), 25 g • Xuan-shen (Radix Scrophulariae, 7 to 35 g), 20 g

119
Formula: Qing-Ying-Tang (0281)

清營湯

Ingredients:

Dan-shen (Radix Salviae Miltiorrhizae, 5 to 10 g), 6 g • Huang-lian (Rhizoma Coptidis, 2 to 12 g), 5 g • Jin-yin-hua (Flos Lonicerae, 7 to 18 g), 15 g • Lian-qiao (Fructus Forsythiae, 5 to 11 g), 6 g • Mai-men-dong (Radix Ophiopogonis, 5 to 11 g), 9 g • Sheng-di (Radix Rehmanniae, 14 to 35 g), 15 g • Xi-jiao (Cornu Rhinoceri, 1 to 2 g), 9 g • Xuan-shen (Radix Scrophulariae, 7 to 35 g), 9 g • Zhu-juan-xin (young bamboo leaf, 3 to 5 g), 3 g

120
Formula: Qing-Zao-Jiu-Fei-Tang (0049)

清燥救肺湯

Ingredients:

E-jiao (Colla Corii Asini, 5 to 11 g), 6 g • Gan-cao (Radix Glycyrrhizae, 2 to 11 g), 3 g • Hu-ma (Semen Sesami, 3 to 10 g), 3g • Mai-men-Dong (Radix Ophiopogonis, 5 to 11 g), 6 g • Pi-pa-ye (Folium Eriobotryae, 5 to 11 g), three leaves • Ren-shen (Radix Ginseng, 1 to 35 g), 10 g • Sang-ye (Folium Mori, 5 to 10 g), 10 g • Shi-gao (Gypsum Fibrosum, 10 to 70 g), 15 g • Xing-ren (Semen Armeniacae Amarae, 5 to 11 g), 10 g

121
Formula: Qing-Zhi-Tang (3365)

清脂湯

Ingredients:

He-shou-wu (Radix Polygoni Multiflori, 11 to 15 g), 12 g • Hei-zhi-ma (Semen Sesami, 4 to 11 g), 12 g • Nu-zhen-zi (Fructus Ligustri Lucidi, 5 to 11 g), 12 g • Sheng-di (Radix Rehimanniae, 14 to 35 g), 12 g • Tu-si-zi (Semen Cuscutae, 5 to 11 g), 15 g • Yin-yang-huo (Herba Epimedii, 4 to 11 g), 10 g • Ze-xie (Rhizoma Alismatis, 7 to 14 g), 15 g

122
Formula: Ren-Shen-Yang-Ying-Tang (0182B)

人參養營湯

Ingredients:

Bai-shao-yao (Radix Paeoniae Alba, 5 to 11 g), 12 g • Bai-zhu (Rhizoma Atractylodis Macrocephalae, 5 to 11 g), 10 g • Chen-pi (Pericarpium Papaveris, 4 to 11 g), 6 g • Dang-gui (Radix Angelicae

Sinensis, 5 to 11 g), 12 g • Dang-shen
(Radix Codonopsis Pilosulae, 11 to 15 g),
10 g • Fu-ling (Poria, 7 to 14 g), 12 g •
Gan-cao (Radix Glycyrrhizae, 2 to 11 g),
3 g • Huang-qi (Radix Astragali Seu
Hedysari, 5 to 40 g), 12 g • Rou-gui
(Cortex Cinnamomi, 1 to 5 g), 6 g • Shu-
di-huang (Radix Rehmanniae Praeparatae,
11 to 18 g), 15 g • Wu-wei-zi (Fructus
Schisandrae, 2 to 4 g), 6 g • Yuan-zhi
(Radix Polygalae, 4 to 11 g), 6 g

123
Formula: Run-Chang-Wan (0159)

潤腸丸

Ingredients:
Dang-gui (Radix Angelicae Sinensis, 5 to
11 g), 10 g • Huo-ma-ren (Fructus
Cannabis, 11 to 17 g), 15 g • Sheng-di
(Radix Rehmanniae, 14 to 35 g), 30 g •
Tao-ren (Semen Persicae, 5 to 11 g), 10 g •
Zhi-qiao (Fructus Aurantii, 4 to 11 g),
10 g

124
Formula: San-Miao-Wan (0392)

三妙丸

Ingredients:
Cang-zhu (Rhizoma Atractylodis
Macrocephalae, 4 to 11 g), 60 g • Huang-
bai (Cortex Phellodendri, 4 to 15 g), 40 g
• Niu-xi (Radix Achyranthis Bidentatae, 5
to 11 g), 20 g

125
Formula: San-Qi-Hong-Teng-Er-Hao-Fang
(3367)

三七紅藤二號方

Ingredients:
Chi-shao-yao (Radix Paeoniae Rubra, 5 to
11 g), 15 g • Chuan-shan-jia (Squama
Manitis, 5 to 11 g), 12 g • Da-xue-teng
(Caulis Sargentodoxae, 10 to 15 g), 15 g •
Dan-shen (Radix Salviae Miltiorrhizae, 5 to

10 g), 15 g • Dang-gui (Radix Angelicae
Sinensis, 5 to 11 g), 15 g • E-zhu
(Rhizoma Zedoariae, 5 to 11 g), 15 g •
Pu-gong-ying (Herba Taraxaci, 7 to 15 g),
15 g • San-qi (Radix Notoginseng, 2 to
10 g), 3 g • Shui-zhi (Hirudo, 2 to 4 g),
6 g • Wu-ling-zhi (Faeces Trogopterorum,
5 to 11 g), 12 g • Xuan-shen (Radix
Scrophulariae, 7 to 35 g), 15 g

126
Formula: San-Qi-Hong-Teng-San-Hao-Fang
(3368)

三七紅藤三號方

Ingredients:
Bai-jiang (Herba Patriniae, 10 to 18 g),
30 g • Chuan-lian-zi (Fructus Meliae
Toosendan, 5 to 11 g), 10 g • Da-qing-ye
(Folium Isatidis, 11 to 18 g), 15 g • Ji-
xue-teng (Caulis Spatholobi, 11 to 35 g),
30 g • Jin-yin-hua (Flos Lonicerae, 7 to
18 g), 15 g • Jin-ying-zi (Fructus Rosae
Laevigatae, 5 to 11 g), 30 g • Qian-cao
(Radix Rubiae, 7 to 11 g), 10 g • San-qi
(Radix Notoginseng, 2 to 10 g), 3 g •
Xiang-fu (Rhizoma Cyperi, 5 to 11 g), 10 g
• Yan-hu-suo (Rhizoma Corydalis, 4 to
11 g), 15 g • Yi-mu-cao (Herba Leonuri,
11 to 36 g), 30 g

127
Formula: San-Qi-Hong-Teng-Yi-Hao-Fang
(3366)

三七紅藤一號方

Ingredients:
Chuan-xiong (Rhizoma Ligustici
Chuanxiong, 2 to 6 g), 6 g • Da-xue-teng
(Caulis Sargentodoxae 10 to 15 g), 30 g •
Dang-gui (Radix Angelicae Sinensis, 5 to
11 g), 15 g • Jin-yin-hua (Flos Lonicerae,
7 to 18 g), 15 g • Mai-men-dong (Radix
Ophiopogonis, 5 to 11 g), 10 g • Mu-dan-
pi (Cortex Moutan Radicis, 5 to 11 g),
10 g • San-qi (Radix Notoginseng, 2 to
10 g), 30 g • Tao-ren (Semen Persicae, 5
to 11 g), 12 g • Xiang-fu (Rhizoma

Cyperi, 5 to 11 g), 12 g • Yi-yi-ren
(Semen Coicis, 11 to 22 g), 30 g

128
Formula: San-Ren-Tang (0107)

三仁湯

Ingredients:
Bai-dou-kou (Fructus Amomi Cardamomi,
2 to 7 g), 10 g • Ban-xia (Rhizoma
Pinelliae, 4 to 12 g), 12 g • Hou-po
(Cortex Magnoliae Officinalis, 4 to 11 g),
12 g • Hua-shi (Talcum, 11 to 15 g), 18 g
• Tong-cao (Medulla Tetrapanacis, 2 to
5 g), 6 g • Xing-ren (Semen Armeniacae
Amarae, 5 to 11 g), 10 g • Yi-yi-ren
(Semen Coicis, 11 to 22 g), 24 g • Zhu-ye
(Folium Bambusae, 4 to 20 g), 6 g

129
Formula: San-Zi-Tang (1885)

三子湯

Ingredients:
Bai-jie-zi (Semen Sinapis Albae, 4 to 11 g),
6 g • Lai-fu-zi (Semen Raphani, 5 to
11 g), 9 g • Zi-su-zi (Fructus Perillae, 5
to 11 g), 9 g

130
Formula: Sang-Ju-Yin (0016)

桑菊飲

Ingredients:
Bo-he (Herba Menthae, 3 to 10 g), 3 g •
Gan-cao (Radix Glycyrrhizae, 2 to 11 g),
3 g • Jie-geng (Radix Platycodi, 2 to 5 g),
9 g • Ju-hua (Flos Chrysanthemi, 4 to
20 g), 12 g • Lian-qiao (Fructus
Forsythiae, 5 to 11 g), 9 g • Lu-gen
(Rhizoma Phragmitis, 15 to 65 g), 15 g •
Sang-ye (Folium Mori, 5 to 10 g), 9 g •
Xing-ren (Semen Armeniacae Amarae, 5 to
11 g), 9 g

131
Formula: Sang-Nu-San-Jia-Tang (3369)

桑女三甲湯

Ingredients:
Bai-shao-yao (Radix Paeoniae Alba, 5 to
11 g), 15 g • Gui-ban (Plastrum
Testudinis, 11 to 30 g), 30 g • Long-gu
(Os Draconis, 11 to 18 g), 30 g • Mu-li
(Concha Ostrae, 11 to 35 g), 30 g • Nu-
zhen-zi (Fructus Ligustri Lucidi, 5 to
11 g), 20 g • Sang-ji-sheng (Ramulus
Loranthi, 11 to 18 g), 20 g • Sheng-di
(Radix Rehmanniae, 14 to 35 g), 15 g •
Tian-dong (Radix Asparagi, 7 to 14 g),
15 g

132
Formula: Sang-Piao-Xiao-San (0326)

桑螵蛸散

Ingredients:
(Use 30 g of each ingredient.)
Chang-pu (Rhizoma Calami, 4 to 7 g) •
Dang-gui (Radix Angelicae Sinensis, 5 to
11 g) • Fu-shen (Buyury with pine root,
11 to 15 g) • Gui-ban (Plastrum
Testudinis, 11 to 30 g) • Long-gu (Os
Draconis, 11 to 18 g) • Ren-shen (Radix
Ginseng, 1 to 35 g) • Sang-piao-xiao
(Ootheca Mantidis, 5 to 11 g) • Yuan-zhi
(Radix Polygalae, 4 to 11 g)

133
Formula: Sang-Xing-Tang (0047)

桑杏湯

Ingredients:
Dan-dou-chi (Semen Sojae Praeparatum, 7
to 14 g), 10 g • Li-pi (Pericarpium
Papaveris/Fructus Papaveris Pyrus, 11 to
18 g), 30 g • Nan-sha-shen (Radix
Adenophorae, 5 to 11 g), 15 g • Sang-ye
(Folium Mori, 5 to 10 g), 15 g • Xing-ren
(Semen Armeniacae Amarae, 5 to 11 g),
10 g • Zhe-bei-mu (Bulbus Fritillariae
Thunbergh, 5 to 11 g), 10 g • Zhi-zi-pi
(Pericarpium Papaveris/Fructus Papaveris
Gardenia, for external use), 12 g

134
Formula: Sha-Shen-Mai-Dong-Tang (0048)

沙參麥冬湯

Ingredients:

Bian-dou (Semen Lalab, 11 to 22 g), 5 g • Gan-cao (Radix Glycyrrhizae, 2 to 11 g), 3 g • Mai-men-dong (Radix Ophiopogonis, 5 to 11 g), 10 g • Nan-sha-shen (Radix Adenophorae, 5 to 11 g), 10 g • Sang-ye (Folium Mori, 5 to 10 g), 6 g • Tian-Hua-fen (Radix Trichosanthis, 10 to 14 g), 6 g • Yu-zhu (Rhizoma Polygonati Odorati, 5 to 11 g), 6 g

135
Formula: *Shao-Fu-Zhu-Yu-Tang (0205)*

少腹逐瘀湯

Ingredients:

Chi-shao-yao (Radix Paeoniae Rubra, 5 to 11 g), 9 g • Chuan-xiong (Rhizoma Ligustici Chuanxiong, 2 to 6 g), 6 g • Dang-gui (Radix Angelicae Sinensis, 5 to 11 g), 9 g • Gan-jiang, pao-jiang, or baked ginger (Rhizoma Zingiberis, 3 to 7 g), 6 g • Mo-yao (Myrrha, 4 to 11 g), 6 g • Pu-huang (Pollen Typhae, 5 to 11 g), 9 g • Rou-gui (Cortex Cinnamomi, 1 to 5 g), 6 g • Wu-ling-zhi (Faeces Trogopterorum, 5 to 11 g), 9 g • Xiao-Hui-Xiang (Fructus Foeniculi, 4 to 11 g), 9 g • Yan-Hu-Suo (Rhizoma Corydalis, 4 to 11 g), 6 g

136
Formula: *Shao-Yao-Tang (0165)*

芍藥湯

Ingredients:

Bing-lang (Semen Areca, 4 to 11 g), 15 g • Chi-shao-yao (Radix Paeoniae Rubra, 5 to 11 g), 15 g • Da-huang (Radix Et Rhizoma Rhei, 4 to 15 g), 12 g • Dang-gui (Radix Angelicae Sinensis, 5 to 11 g), 6 g • Gan-cao (Radix Glycyrrhizae, 2 to 11 g), 3 g • Huang-lian (Rhizoma Coptidis, 2 to 12 g), 10 g • Huang-qin (Radix Scutellariae, 4 to 15 g), 12 g • Mu-xiang (Radix Aucklandiae/Radix Saussureae, 2 to 6 g), 10 g • Rou-gui (Cortex Cinnamomi, 1 to 5 g), 6 g

137
Formula: *She-Gan-Ma-Huang-Tang (0026)*

射干麻黃湯

Ingredients:

Ban-xia (Rhizoma Pinelliae, 4 to 12 g), 12 g • Da-zao (Fructus Ziziphi Jujubae, 7 to 18 g), 9 g • Kuan-dong-hua (Flos Farfarae, 5 to 11 g), 12 g • Ma-huang (Herba Ephedrae, 5 to 10 g), 9 g • She-gan (Rhizoma Belamcandae, 2 to 5 g), 9 g • Sheng-jiang (Rhizoma Zingiberis Recens, 4 to 10 g), 9 g • Wu-wei-zi (Fructus Schisandrae, 2 to 4 g), 6 g • Xi-xin (Herba Asari, 1 to 4 g), 6 g • Zi-wan (Radix Asteris, 5 to 11 g), 9 g

138
Formula: *Shen-Fu-Long-Mu-Jiu-Ni-Tang (1898)*

參附龍骨牡蠣救逆湯

Ingredients:

Fu-zi (Radix Aconiti Praeparata, 4 to 11 g), 11 g • Long-gu (Os Draconis, 11 to 18 g), 18 g • Mu-li (Concha Ostrae, 11 to 35 g), 35 g • Ren-shen (Radix Ginseng, 1 to 35 g), 35 g

139
Formula: *Shen-Fu-Tang (0318)*

參附湯

Ingredients:

Fu-zi (Radix Aconiti Praeparata, 4 to 11 g), 15 to 60 g • Ren-shen (Radix Ginseng, 1 to 35 g), 15 g

140
Formula: *Shen-Huang-Gan-Qi-Tang (3370)*

參黃甘杞湯

Ingredients:

Dang-shen (Radix Codonopsis Pilosulae, 11 to 15 g), 15 g • Gan-cao (Radix

Glycyrrhizae, 2 to 11 g), 11 g • Gou-qi-zi (Fructus Lych, 5 to 11 g), 11 g • Huang-jing (Rhizoma Polygonati, 11 to 15 g), 15 g

141
Formula: *Shen-Ling-Bai-Zhu-San* (0081)

參苓白术散

Ingredients:
Bai-zhu (Rhizoma Atractylodis Macrocephalae, 5 to 11 g), 10 g • Bian-dou (Semen Lalab, 11 to 22 g), 12 g • Chen-pi (Pericarpium Papaveris, 4 to 11 g), 12 g • Dang-shen (Radix Codonopsis Pilosulae, 11 to 15 g), 15 g • Fu-ling (Poria, 7 to 14 g), 15 g • Gan-cao (Radix Glycyrrhizae, 2 to 11 g), 3 g • Jie-geng (Radix Platycodi, 2 to 5 g), 6 g • Lian-zi (Semen Nelumbinis, 7 to 18 g), 15 g • Sha-ren (Fructus Amomi, 2 to 7 g), 9 g • Shan-yao (Rhizoma Dioscoreae, 10 to 20 g), 15 g • Yi-yi-ren (Semen Coicis, 11 to 22 g), 24 g

142
Formula: *Shen-Qi-Si-Wu-Tang* (3371)

參芪四物湯

Ingredients:
Bai-shao-yao (Radix Paeoniae Alba, 5 to 11 g), 10 g • Bai-zhu (Rhizoma Atractylodis Macrocephalae, 5 to 11 g), 10 g • Chuan-xiong (Rhizoma Ligustici Chuanxiong, 2 to 6 g), 6 g • Dang-gui (Radix Angelicae Sinensis, 5 to 11 g), 10 g • Dang-shen (Radix Codonopsis Pilosulae, 11 to 15 g), 10 g • Gan-cao (Radix Glycyrrhizae, 2 to 11 g), 6 g • Huang-qi (Radix Astragali Seu Hedysari, 3 to 40 g), 30 g • Shu-di-huang (Radix Rehmanniae Praeparatae, 11 to 18 g), 12 g • Suan-zao-ren (Semen Ziziphi Spinosae, 7 to 18 g), 12 g • Wu-wei-zi (Fructus Schisandrae, 2 to 4 g), 10 g

143
Formula: *Shen-Qi-Wan* (0331)

腎氣丸

Ingredients:
Fu-ling (Poria, 7 to 14 g), 90 g • Fu-zi (Radix Aconiti Praeparata, 4 to 11 g), 30 g • Gan-di (Dried Radix Rehmanniae, 11 to 18 g), 240 g • Gui-zhi (Ramulus Cinnamomi, 2 to 10 g), 30 g • Mu-dan-pi (Cortex Moutan Radicis, 5 to 11 g), 90 g • Shan-yao (Rhizoma Dioscoreae, 10 to 20 g), 120 g • Shan-zhu-yu (Fructus Corni, 5 to 11 g), 120 g • Ze-xie (Rhizoma Alismatis, 7 to 14 g), 90 g

Instructions: Grind into powder to make tablets with honey. Take 9 g of tablets one to two times daily, with warm or lightly salted water. Use reduced quantities of ingredients if decoction is done.

144
Formula: *Shen-Tong-Zhu-Yu-Tang* (1084)

身痛逐瘀湯

Ingredients:
Chuan-xiong (Rhizoma Ligustici Chuanxiong, 2 to 6 g), 6 g • Dang-gui (Radix Angelicae Sinensis, 5 to 11 g), 9 g • Di-long (Lumbricus, 5 to 11 g), 6 g • Gan-cao (Radix Glycyrrhizae, 2 to 11 g), 6 g • Hong-hua (Flos Carthami, 4 to 7 g), 9 g • Mo-yao (Myrrha, 4 to 11 g), 6 g • Niu-xi (Radix Achyranthis Bidentatae, 5 to 11 g), 9 g • Qiang-huo (Rhizoma Seu Radix Notopterygii, 4 to 10 g), 3 g • Qin-jiao (Radix Gentianae Macrophyllae 4 to 11 g), 3 g • Tao-ren (Semen Persicae, 5 to 11 g), 9 g • Wu-ling-zhi (Faeces Trogopterorum, 5 to 11 g), 6 g • Xiang-fu (Rhizoma Cyperi, 5 to 11 g), 3 g

145
Formula: *Shen-Zhe-Zhen-Qi-Tang* (1839)

參赭鎮氣湯

Ingredients:
Bai-shao-yao (Radix Paeoniae Alba, 5 to 11 g), 12 g • Dai-zhe-shi (Ocherum Rubrum, 1 to 35 g), 18 g • Dang-shen (Radix Codonopsis Pilosulae, 11 to 15 g),

12 g • *Long-gu (Os Draconis, 11 to 18 g),* 18 g • *Mu-li (Concha Ostrae, 11 to 35 g),* 18 g • *Qian-shi (Semen Euryales, 7 to 11 g),* 15 g • *Shan-yao (Rhizoma Dioscoreae, 10 to 20 g),* 15 g • *Shan-zhu-yu (Fructus Corni, 5 to 11 g),* 18 g • *Zi-su-zi Fructus Perillae, 5 to 11 g),* 6 g

146
Formula: *Shen-Zhuo-Tang (0617)*

腎著湯

Ingredients:
Bai-zhu (Rhizoma Atractylodis Macrocephalae, 5 to 11 g), 6 g • *Fu-ling (Poria, 7 to 14 g),* 9 g • *Gan-cao (Radix Glycyrrhizae, 2 to 11 g),* 3 g • *Gan-Jiang (Rhizoma Zingiberis, 3 to 7 g),* 6 g

147
Formula: *Sheng-Mai-San (0315)*

生脈散

Ingredients:
Mai-men-dong (Radix Ophiopogonis, 5 to 11 g), 9 g • *Ren-shen (Radix Ginseng, 1 to 35 g),* 15 g • *Wu-wei-zi (Fructus Schisandrae, 2 to 4 g),* 6 g

148
Formula: *Shi-Gao-Zhi-Mu-Jia-Ren-Shen-Tang (0065G)*

石膏知母加人參湯

Ingredients:
Gan-cao (Radix Glycyrrhizae, 2 to 11 g), 6 g • *Jing-mi (polished rice, flexible quantity),* 9 g • *Ren-shen (Radix Ginseng, 1 to 35 g),* 10 g • *Shi-gao (Gypsum Fibrosum, 10 to 70 g),* 15 to 60 g • *Zhi-mu (Rhizoma Anemarrhenae, 4 to 15 g),* 12 g

149
Formula: *Shi-Pi-Yin (0132)*

實脾飲

Ingredients:
Bai-zhu (Rhizoma Atractylodis Macrocephalae, 5 to 11 g), 10 g • *Bing-lang (Semen Areca, 4 to 11 g),* 15 g • *Cao-Guo (Fructus Tsaoko, 2 to 5 g),* 10 g • *Fu-ling (Poria, 7 to 14 g),* 15 g • *Fu-zi (Radix Aconiti Praeparata, 4 to 11 g),* 15 g • *Gan-cao (Radix Glycyrrhizae, 2 to 11 g),* 3 g • *Gan-Jiang (Rhizoma Zingiberis, 3 to 7 g),* 10 g • *Hou-po (Cortex Magnoliae Officinalis, 4 to 11 g),* 12 g • *Mu-gua (Fructus Chaenomelis, 5 to 11 g),* 12 g • *Mu-xiang (Radix Aucklandiae/Radix Saussureae, 2 to 6 g),* 6 g

150
Formula: *Shi-Quan-Da-Bu-Wan (0182A)*

十全大補丸

Ingredients:
Bai-shao-yao (Radix Paeoniae Alba, 5 to 11 g), 12 g • *Bai-zhu (Rhizoma Atractylodis Macrocephalae, 5 to 11 g),* 10 g • *Chuan-xiong (Rhizoma Ligustici Chuanxiong, 2 to 6 g),* 6 g • *Dang-gui (Radix Angelicae Sinensis, 5 to 11 g),* 12 g • *Dang-shen (Radix Codonopsis Pilosulae, 11 to 15 g),* 10 g • *Fu-ling (Poria, 7 to 14 g),* 12 g • *Gan-cao (Radix Glycyrrhizae, 2 to 11 g),* 3 g • *Huang-qi (Radix Astragali Seu Hedysari, 5 to 40 g),* 12 g • *Rou-gui (Cortex Cinnamomi, 1 to 5 g),* 4 g • *Shu-di-huang (Radix Rehmanniae Praeparatae, 11 to 18 g),* 15 g

151
Formula: *Shi-Xiao-San (0201)*

失笑散

Ingredients:
(Use equal quantities of both ingredients.)
Pu-huang (Pollen Typhae, 5 to 11 g) • *Wu-ling-zhi (Faeces Trogopterorum, 5 to 11 g)*
Instructions: Grind into powder, and take 6 g of powder twice daily.

152
Formula: *Shu-Zao-Yin-Zi* (0134C)

疏鑿飲子

Ingredients:
(Use 8 g of each ingredient.)
Bing-lang (Semen Areca, 4 to 11 g) • *Chi-xiao-dou (Semen Phaseoli, 11 to 18 g)* •
Da-fu-pi (Pericarpium Arecae, 5 to 18 g) •
Fu-ling-pi (Poria, outer skin, 10 to 18 g) •
*Jiang-pi (Exocarpium Zingiberis (Recens,
15 to 45 g)* • *Jiao-mu (Semen Zanthoxyli,
8 g)* • *Mu-tong (Caulis Aristolochiae, 4 to
8 g)* • *Qiang-huo (Rhizoma Seu Radix
Notopterygii, 4 to 10 g)* • *Qin-jiao (Radix
Gentianae Macrophyllae, 4 to 11 g)* •
Shang-lu (Radix Phytolaccae, 2 to 5 g) •
Ze-xie (Rhizoma Alismatis, 7 to 14 g)

153
Formula: *Si-Hai-Shu-Yu-Wan* (0993)

四海舒郁丸

Ingredients:
*Chen-pi (Pericarpium Citri Reticulatae
Viride, 4 to 11 g), 9 g* • *Ge-li-fen (Clam-
Shell Powder, 3 to 10 g), 9 g* • *Hai-dai
(Seaweed, 5 to 10 g), 60 g* • *Hai-piao-
xiao (Os Sepiellae Seu Sepiae, 5 to 11 g),
60 g* • *Hai-zao (Sargassum, 5 to 11 g),
60 g* • *Kun-bu (Thallus Laminariae Seu
Eckloniae, 5 to 11 g), 60 g* • *Qing-mu-
xiang (Radix Aristolochiae, 4 to 11 g),
15 g*
Instructions: Grind into powder, and
take 6 g of powder twice daily.

154
Formula: *Si-Jun-Zi-Tang* (0080)

四君子湯

Ingredients:
*Bai-zhu (Rhizoma Atractylodis
Macrocephalae, 5 to 11 g), 10 g* • *Fu-ling
(Poria, 7 to 14 g), 12 g* • *Gan-cao (Radix
Glycyrrhizae, 2 to 11 g), 3 g* • *Ren-shen
(Radix Ginseng, 1 to 35 g), 15 g*

155
Formula: *Si-Ni-Jia-Ren-Shen-Tang* (0317C)

四逆加人參湯

Ingredients:
*Fu-zi (Radix Aconiti Praeparata, 4 to
11 g), 15 to 30 g* • *Gan-cao, zhi-gan-cao
(Radix Glycyrrhizae, 2 to 11 g), 12 g* •
*Gan-jiang (Rhizoma Zingiberis, 3 to 7 g),
9 g* • *Ren-shen (Radix Ginseng, 1 to 35 g),
flexible quantity*

156
Formula: *Si-Ni-San* (0178)

四逆散

Ingredients:
Chai-hu (Radix Bupleuri, 4 to 16 g), 12 g
• *Chi-shao-yao (Radix Paeoniae Rubra, 5 to
11 g), 30 to 100 g* • *Gan-cao (Radix
Glycyrrhizae, 2 to 11 g), 6 g* • *Zhi-shi
(Fructus Auranth Immaturus, 4 to 7 g),
12 g*
Instructions: Grind into powder, and
take 6 g of powder twice daily.

157
Formula: *Si-Ni-Tang* (0317)

四逆湯

Ingredients:
*Fu-zi (Radix Aconiti Praeparata, 4 to
11 g), 15 to 30 g* • *Gan-cao, zhi-gan-cao
(Radix Glycyrrhizae, 2 to 11 g), 12 g* •
*Gan-jiang (Rhizoma Zingiberis, 3 to 7 g),
9 g*

158
Formula: *Si-Shen-Wan* (0169)

四神丸

Ingredients:
*Bu-gu-zhi (Fructus Psoraleae, 4 to 11 g),
120 g* • *Rou-dou-kou (Semen Myristicae, 2
to 8 g), 60 g* • *Wu-wei-zi (Fructus
Schisandrae, 2 to 4 g), 60 g* • *Wu-zhu-yu
(Fructus Euodiae, 2 to 7 g), 30 g*

Instructions: Grind into powder to make tablets, and take 6 g of tablets each time.

159

Formula: *Si-Sheng-Wan* (0984)

四生丸

Ingredients:

Ai-ye (Folium Artemisiae Argyi, 4 to 11 g), 60 g • *Ce-bai-ye (Caumen Biotae, 7 to 14 g),* 60 g • *He-ye (Folium Nelumbinis, 4 to 11 g),* 60 g • *Sheng-di (Radix Rehmanniae, 14 to 35 g),* 60 g

Instructions: Grind into powder, and take 6 g of powder twice daily.

160

Formula: *Si-Wu-Tang* (0196)

四物湯

Ingredients:

Bai-shao-yao (Radix Paeoniae Alba, 5 to 11 g), 24 g • *Chuan-xiong (Rhizoma Ligustici Chuanxiong, 2 to 6 g),* 3 g • *Dang-gui (Radix Angelicae Sinensis, 5 to 11 g),* 12 g • *Shu-di-huang (Radix Rehmanniae Praeparatae, 11 to 18 g),* 20 g

161

Formula: *Su-He-Xiang-Wan* (0292)

蘇合香丸

Ingredients:

An-xi-xiang (Benzoinum, 0.3 to 2 g), 60 g • *Bai-zhu (Rhizoma Atractylodis Macrocephalae, 5 to 11 g),* 60 g • *Bi-bo (Fructus, Piperis Longi, 2 to 4 g),* 60 g • *Bing-pian (Borneol, 0.2 to 0.3 g),* 60 g • *Chen-xiang (Lignum Aquilariae Resinatum, 1 to 4 g),* 60 g • *Ding-xiang (Flos Caryophylli, 1 to 4 g),* 60 g • *He-zi (Fructus Chebulae, 2 to 5 g),* 60 g • *Qing-mu-xiang (Radix Aristolochiae, 4 to 11 g),* 60 g • *Ru-xiang (Mastix/Resina, 4 to 11 g),* 30 g • *She-xiang (Moschus, 0.01 to 0.03 g),* 60 g • *Su-he-xiang (Styrax*

Liquidus oil, 0.5 g), 30 g • *Tan-xiang (Lignum Santali Album, 2 to 4 g),* 60 g • *Xi-jiao (Cornu Rhinoceri, 1 to 2 g),* 60 g • *Xiang-fu (Rhizoma Cyperi, 5 to 11 g),* 60 g • *Zhu-sha (Cinnabaris, 0.3 to 1 g),* 60 g

Instructions: Grind into powder to make tablets, and take half to one tablet or 3 g each time.

162

Formula: *Suo-Niao-Wan* (0334)

Ingredients: (Use equal quantities of both ingredients.)

縮尿丸

Wu-yao (Radix Linderae, 5 to 10 g) • *Yi-zhi-ren (Fructus Zigiberis Nigri, 4 to 11 g)*

Instructions: Decoct Shan-Yao powder in wine, and grind the ingredients into powder. Use the decoction to make tablets, with each one the size of a Chinese parasol seed, called wu-tong-zi. Take 6 g of tablets each time.

163

Formula: *Tai-Wu-Shen-Zhu-San* (2164)

太元神术散

Ingredients:

Cang-zhu (Rhizoma Atractylodis, 4 to 11 g), 30 g • *Chen-pi (Pericarpium Citri Reticulatae, 4 to 11 g),* 30 g • *Da-zao (Fructus Ziziphi Jujubae, 7 to 18 g),* 40 g • *Hou-po (Cortex Magnoliae Officinalis, 4 to 11 g),* 30 g • *Huo-xiang (Herba Agastachis, 5 to 11 g),* 30 g • *Sheng-jiang (Rhizoma Zingiberis Recens, 4 to 10 g),* 35 g • *Shi-chang-pu (Rhizoma Acori Graminei, 2 to 5 g),* 20 g

Instructions: Grind into powder, and take 9 g of powder twice daily.

164

Formula: *Tao-Hong-Si-Wu-Tang* (0196G)

桃紅四物湯

Ingredients:

Bai-shao-yao (Radix Paeoniae Alba, 5 to 11 g), 24 g • *Chuan-xiong (Rhizoma*

Ligustici Chuanxiong, 2 to 6 g), 3 g •
Dang-gui (Radix Angelicae Sinensis, 5 to
11 g), 12 g • Hong-hua (Flos Carthami, 4
to 7 g), 3 g • Shu-di-huang (Radix
Rehmanniae Praeparatae, 11 to 18 g), 20 g
• Tao-ren (Semen Persicae, 5 to 11 g), 3 g

165
Formula: Tao-Ren-Fu-Su-Fang (3373)

桃仁復蘇方

Ingredients:
Da-huang (Radix Et Rhizoma Rhei, 4 to
15 g), 10 g • Gan-cao (Radix
Glycyrrhizae, 2 to 11 g), 6 g • Gui-zhi
(Ramulus Cinnamomi, 2 to 10 g), 10 g •
Mu-li (Concha Ostrae, 11 to 35 g), 30 g •
Shi-chang-pu (Rhizoma Acori Graminei, 2
to 5 g), 10 g • Tao-ren (Semen Persicae, 5
to 11 g), 10 g • Wu-gong (Scolopendra,
0.1 to 0.2 g), 10 g • Xuan-ming-fen
(Mirabilitum Dehydratum, 4 to 11 g), 10 g
• Yuan-zhi (Radix Polygalae, 4 to 11 g),
10 g • Zhu-sha (Cinnabaris, 0.3 to 1 g),
15 g

166
Formula: Tian-Wang-Bu-Xin-Dan (0920)

天王補心丹

Ingredients:
Bai-zi-ren (Semen Biotae, 4 to 11 g), 30 g
• Dan-shen (Radix Salviae Miltiorrhizae, 5
to 10 g), 15 g • Dang-gui (Radix
Angelicae Sinensis, 5 to 11 g), 30 g • Fu-
ling (Poria, 7 to 14 g), 15 g • Jie-geng
(Radix Platycodi, 2 to 5 g), 15 g • Mai-
men-dong (Radix Ophiopogonis, 5 to 11 g),
30 g • Ren-shen (Radix Ginseng, 1 to
35 g), 15 g • Sheng-di (Radix Rehmanniae,
14 to 35 g), 120 g • Suan-zao-ren Semen
Ziziphi Spinosae, 7 to 18 g), 30 g • Tian-
dong (Radix Asparagi, 7 to 14 g), 30 g •
Wu-wei-zi (Fructus Schisandrae, 2 to 4 g),
30 g • Xuan-shen (Radix Scrophulariae, 7
to 35 g), 15 g • Yuan-zhi (Radix
Polygalae, 4 to 11 g), 15 g • Zhu-sha
(Cinnabaris, 0.3 to 1 g), 1.5 g

Instructions: Grind into powder to make
tablets with honey, and take 9 g of
tablets twice daily.

167
Formula: Tong-Guan-Wan (0732)

通關丸

Ingredients:
Huang-bai (Cortex Phellodendri, 4 to
15 g), 30 g • Rou-gui (Cortex Cinnamomi,
1 to 5 g), 1.5 g • Zhi-mu (Rhizoma
Anemarrhenae, 4 to 15 g), 30 g

168
Formula: Tong-Qiao-Huo-Xue-Tang (0214)

通竅活血湯

Ingredients:
Chi-shao-yao (Radix Paeoniae Rubra, 5 to
11 g), 9 g • Chuan-xiong (Rhizoma
Ligustici Chuanxiong, 2 to 6 g), 9 g • Da-
zao (Fructus Ziziphi Jujubae, 7 to 18 g),
9 g • Hong-hua (Flos Carthami, 4 to 7 g),
9 g • She-xiang (Moschus, 0.01 to 0.03 g),
0.3 g • Sheng-jiang (Rhizoma Zingiberis
Recens, 4 to 10 g), 9 g • Tao-ren (Semen
Persicae, 5 to 11 g), 9 g
Old green onion, three roots

169
Formula: Tong-Xie-Yao-Fang

痛瀉要方

Ingredients:
Bai-shao-yao (Radix Paeoniae Alba, 5 to
11 g), 20 g • Bai-zhu (Rhizoma
Atractylodis Macrocephalae, 5 to 11 g),
12 g • Chen-pi (Pericarpium Papaveris, 4
to 11 g), 9 g • Fang-feng (Radix
Ledebouriellae, 5 to 10 g), 6 g

170
Formula: Wei-Jing-Tang (0037)

葦莖湯

Ingredients:

Dong-gua-ren (Semen Benincasae, 3 to 14 g), 24 g • Lu-jing (Caulis Phragmitis, 15 to 35 g), 60 to 120 g • Tao-ren (Semen Persicae, 5 to 11 g), 9 g • Yi-yi-ren (Semen Coicis, 11 to 22 g), 30 g

171
Formula: Wei-Ling-Tang (0117F)

胃苓湯

Ingredients:

Bai-zhu (Rhizoma Atractylodis Macrocephalae, 5 to 11 g), 9 g • Cang-zhu (Rhizoma Atractylodis Macrocephalae, 4 to 11 g), 10 g • Chen-pi (Pericarpium Papaveris, 4 to 11 g), 10 g • Fu-ling (Poria, 7 to 14 g), 12 g • Gan-cao (Radix Glycyrrhizae, 2 to 11 g), 3 g • Gui-zhi (Ramulus Cinnamomi, 2 to 10 g), 9 g • Hou-po (Cortex Magnoliae Officinalis, 4 to 11 g), 10 g • Ze-xie (Rhizoma Alismatis, 7 to 14 g), 15 g • Zhu-ling (Polyporus Umbellatus, 7 to 14 g), 12 g

172
Formula: Wen-Dan-Tang (0124)

溫膽湯

Ingredients:

Ban-xia (Rhizoma Pinelliae, 4 to 12 g), 12 g • Chen-pi (Pericarpium Papaveris, 4 to 11 g), 10 g • Fu-ling (Poria, 7 to 14 g), 12 g • Gan-cao (Radix Glycyrrhizae, 2 to 11 g), 3 g • Zhi-shi (Fructus Aurantii Immaturus, 4 to 7 g), 6 g • Zhu-ru (Caulis Bambusae in Taeniam, 5 to 11 g), 10 g

173
Formula: Wen-Fei-Zhi-Liu-Dan (0807)

溫肺止流丹

Ingredients:

Gan-cao (Radix Glycyrrhizae, 2 to 11 g), 4 g • He-zi (Fructus Chebulae, 2 to 5 g), 4 g • Jie-geng (Radix Platycodi, 2 to 5 g),

12 g • Jing-jie (Herba Schizonepetae, 5 to 10 g), 2 g • Ren-shen (Radix Ginseng, 1 to 35 g), 2 g • Xi-xin (Herba Asari, 1 to 4 g), 2 g

174
Formula: Wen-Pi-Tang (0158)

溫脾湯

Ingredients:

Da-Huang (Radix Et Rhizoma Rhei, 4 to 15 g), 12 g • Fu-zi (Radix Aconiti Praeparata, 4 to 11 g), 15 g • Gan-cao (Radix Glycyrrhizae, 2 to 11 g), 6 g • Gan-jiang (Rhizoma Zingiberis, 3 to 7 g), 10 g • Ren-shen (Radix Ginseng, 1 to 35 g), 6 g

175
Formula: Wu-Hu-Zhui-Feng-San (0250)

五虎追風散

Ingredients:

Chan-tui (Periostracum Cicadae, 2 to 5 g), 30 g • Jiang-can (Bombyx Batryticatus, 5 to 11 g), seven pieces • Quan-xie (Scorpio, 2 to 5 g), seven insects • Tian-ma (Rhizoma Gastrodiae, 4 to 11 g), 6 g • Tian-nan-xing (Rhizoma Arisaematis, 2.5 to 5 g), 6 g • Zhu-sha (Cinnabaris, 0.3 to 1 g), 1.5 g

Instructions: Decoct the herbs; then strain and mix with 60 g of yellow wine. Drink 1.5 g of Zhu-Sha first, before drinking the decoction. Take once daily for three days.

176
Formula: Wu-Ling-San (0348)

五苓散

Ingredients:

Bai-zhu (Rhizoma Atractylodis Macrocephalae, 5 to 11 g), 9 g • Fu-ling (Poria, 7 to 14 g), 12 g • Gui-zhi (Ramulus Cinnamomi, 2 to 10 g), 9 g • Ze-xie (Rhizoma Alismatis, 7 to 14 g),

15 g • Zhu-ling (Polyporus Umbellatus, 7 to 14 g), 12 g

177
Formula: *Wu-Mo-Yin-Zi* (0433)

五磨飲子

Ingredients:
(Use equal quantities of all ingredients.)
Bing-lang (Semen Areca, 4 to 11 g) •
Chen-xiang (Lignum Aquilariae Resinatum, 1 to 4 g) • *Wu-Yao (Radix Linderae, 5 to 10 g)* • *Zhi-shi (Fructus Aurantii Immaturus, 4 to 7 g)*
Instructions: Grind into powder, and take 6 g of powder twice daily.

178
Formula: *Wu-Pi-Yin* (0130)

五皮飲

Ingredients:
(Use equal quantities of all ingredients.)
Chen-pi (Pericarpium Papaveris, 4 to 11 g) • *Da-fu-pi (Pericarpium Papaveris/Fructus Papaveris Arecae, 5 to 18 g)* • *Fu-ling-pi (Poria, outer skin, 10 to 18 g)* • *Sang-bai-pi (Cortex Mori Radicis, 5 to 11 g)* • *Sheng-jiang (Rhizoma Zingiberis Recens, 4 to 10 g)*

179
Formula: *Wu-Tou-Tang* (0465)

烏頭湯

Ingredients:
Bai-shao-yao (Radix Paeoniae Alba, 5 to 11 g), 9 g • *Chuan-wu (Radix Aconiti, 1.5 to 5 g), 15 g* • *Gan-cao (Radix Glycyrrhizae, 2 to 11 g), 9 g* • *Huang-qi (Radix Astragali Seu Hedysari 5 to 40 g), 15 g* • *Ma-Huang (Herba Ephedrae, 5 to 10 g), 8 g*

180
Formula: *Wu-Wei-Di-Huang-Tang* (2157)

五味地黃湯

Ingredients:
Gou-qi-zi (Fructus Lych, 5 to 11 g), 10 g •
Ren-shen (Radix Ginseng, 1 to 35 g), 24 g • *Shan-zhu-yu (Fructus Corni, 5 to 11 g), 10 g* • *Shu-di-huang (Radix Rehmanniae Praeparatae, 11 to 18 g), 15 g* • *Tian-dong (Radix Asparagi, 7 to 14 g), 10 g*

181
Formula: *Wu-Zhu-Yu-Tang* (0185)

吳茱萸湯

Ingredients:
Da-zao (Fructus Ziziphi Jujubae, 7 to 18 g), 9 g • *Ren-shen (Radix Ginseng, 1 to 35 g), 9 g* • *Sheng-jiang (Rhizoma Zingiberis Recens, 4 to 10 g), 9 g* • *Wu-zhu-yu (Fructus Euodiae, 2 to 7 g), 9 g*

182
Formula: *Wu-Zi-Yan-Zong-Wan* (0915)

五子衍宗丸

Ingredients:
Che-qian-zi (Semen Plantaginis, 4 to 11 g), 60 g • *Fu-pen-zi (Fructus Rubi, 5 to 11 g), 120 g* • *Gou-qi-zi (Fructus Lych, 5 to 11 g), 240 g* • *Tu-si-zi (Semen Cuscutae, 5 to 11 g), 240 g* • *Wu-wei-zi (Fructus Schisandrae, 2 to 4 g), 30 g*
Instructions: Grind into powder to make tablets with honey, and take 9 g of tablets twice daily.

183
Formula: *Xi-Gan-San* (3376)

洗肝散

Ingredients:
(Use equal quantities of all ingredients.)
Da-huang (Radix Et Rhizoma Rhei, 4 to 15 g), 50 g • *Dang-gui (Radix Angelicae Sinensis, 5 to 11 g), 50 g* • *Fang-feng (Radix Ledebouriellae, 5 to 10 g), 50 g* • *Huang-qin (Radix Scutellariae, 4 to 15 g), 50 g* • *Qiang-huo (Rhizoma Seu Radix Notopterygii, 4 to 10 g), 50 g* • *Xuan-shen (Radix Scrophulariae, 7 to 35 g), 50 g*

Instructions: Grind into powder, and take 9 g of powder twice daily.

184
Formula: *Xi-Jiao-Di-Huang-Tang* (0285)

犀角地黃湯

Ingredients:
Chi-shao-yao (Radix Paeoniae Rubra, 5 to 11 g), 12 g • Mu-dan-pi (Cortex Moutan Radicis, 5 to 11 g), 9 g • Sheng-di (Radix Rehmanniae, 14 to 35 g), 30 g • Xi-jiao (Cornu Rhinoceri, 1 to 2 g), 9 g

185
Formula: *Xi-Xin-Tang* (1147)

細辛湯

Ingredients:
Chong-wei-zi (Fructus Leonuri, 5 to 11 g), 60 g • Da-huang (Radix Et Rhizoma Rhei, 4 to 15 g), 30 g • Fang-feng (Radix Ledebouriellae, 5 to 10 g), 60 g • Jie-geng (Radix Platycodi, 2 to 5 g), 60 g • Ling-yang-jiao (Cornu Antelopis, 1 to 1.5 g), 10 g • Xi-xin (Herba Asari, 1 to 4 g), 60 g • Xuan-shen (Radix Scrophulariae, 7 to 35 g), 60 g • Zhi-mu (Rhizoma Anemarrhenae, 4 to 15 g), 60 g
Instructions: Grind into powder, and take 6 g of powder twice daily.

186
Formula: *Xiang-Sha-Liu-Jun-Zi-Tang* (0080D)

香砂六君子湯

Ingredients:
Bai-zhu (Rhizoma Atractylodis Macrocephalae, 5 to 11 g), 10 g • Ban-xia (Rhizoma Pinelliae, 4 to 12 g), 7 g • Chen-pi (Pericarpium Papaveris, 4 to 11 g), 7 g • Fu-ling (Poria, 7 to 14 g), 12 g • Gan-cao (Radix Glycyrrhizae, 2 to 11 g), 3 g • Mu-xiang (Radix Aucklandiae/Radix Saussureae, 2 to 6 g), 7 g • Ren-shen (Radix Ginseng, 1 to 35 g), 15 g • Sha-ren (Fructus Amomi, 2 to 7 g), 5 g

187
Formula: *Xiao-Ban-Xia-Jia-Fu-Ling-Tang* (0093A)

小半夏加茯苓湯

Ingredients:
Ban-xia (Rhizoma Pinelliae, 4 to 12 g), 15 g • Fu-ling (Poria, 7 to 14 g), 9 g • Sheng-jiang (Rhizoma Zingiberis Recens, 4 to 10 g), 9 g

188
Formula: *Xiao-Ban-Xia-Tang* (0093)

小半夏湯

Ingredients:
Ban-xia (Rhizoma Pinelliae, 4 to 12 g), 15 g • Sheng-jiang (Rhizoma Zingiberis Recens, 4 to 10 g), 9 g

189
Formula: *Xiao-Chai-Hu-Tang* (0255)

小柴胡湯

Ingredients:
Ban-xia-(Rhizoma Pinelliae, 4 to 12 g), 9 g • Chai-hu (Radix Bupleuri, 4 to 16 g), 15 g • Da-Zao (Fructus Ziziphi Jujubae, 7 to 18 g), four dates • Gan-cao (Radix Glycyrrhizae, 2 to 11 g), 3 g • Huang-qin (Radix Scutellariae, 4 to 15 g), 12 g • Ren-shen (Radix Ginseng, 1 to 35 g), 9 g • Sheng-Jiang (Rhizoma Zingiberis Recens, 4 to 10 g), 9 g

190
Formula: *Xiao-Feng-San* (0014)

消風散

Ingredients:
Bo-he-(Herba Menthae, 3 to 10 g), 9 g • Chan-tui (Periostracum Cicadae, 2 to 5 g), 9 g • Chen-pi (Pericarpium Citri Reticulatae, 4 to 11 g), 6 g • Chuan-xiong (Rhizoma Ligustici Chuanxiong, 2 to 6 g), 9 g • Dang-shen (Radix Codonopsis

Pilosulae, 11 to 15 g), 20 g • Fang-feng
(Radix Ledebouriellae, 5 to 10 g), 9 g •
Fu-ling (Poria, 7 to 14 g), 9 g • Hou-po
(Cortex Magnoliae Officinalis, 4 to 11 g),
6 g • Jiang-can (Bombyx Batryticatus, 5 to
11 g), 9 g • Jing-jie (Herba Schizonepetae,
5 to 10 g), 9 g • Qiang-huo (Rhizoma Seu
Radix Notopterygii Notopterygii, 4 to 10 g),
9 g

191
Formula: Xiao-Ji-Yin-Zi (0353)

小薊飲子

Ingredients:
Dan-zhu-ye (Herba Lophatheri, 4 to 11 g),
9 g • Dang-gui (Radix Angelicae Sinensis,
5 to 11 g), 6 g • Gan-cao (Radix
Glycyrrhizae, 2 to 11 g), 3 g • Hua-shi
(Talcum, 11 to 15 g), 15 g • Mu-tong
(Caulis Aristolochiae, 4 to 8 g), 12 g •
Ou-jie (Nodus Nelumbinis Rhizomatis, 5 to
11 g), 15 g • Pu-huang (Pollen Typhae, 5
to 11 g), 9 g • Sheng-di (Radix
Rehmanniae, 14 to 35 g), 15 g • Xiao-ji
(Herba Cephalanoploris, 6 to 11 g), 15 g •
Zhi-zi (Fructus Gardeniae, 7 to 16 g), 9 g

192
Formula: Xiao-Ke-Fang (0704)

消渴方

Ingredients:
Huang-lian (Rhizoma Coptidis, 2 to 12 g),
8 g • Sheng-di (Radix Rehmanniae, 14 to
35 g), 30 g • Tian-hua-fen (Radix
Trichosanthis, 10 to 14 g), 12 g
Instructions: Grind into powder, and
take 9 g of powder with honey twice
daily.

193
Formula: Xiao-Yao-San (0229)

逍遙散

Ingredients:
Bai-shao-yao (Radix Paeoniae Alba, 5 to
11 g), 30 g • Bai-zhu (Rhizoma

Atractylodis Macrocephalae, 5 to 11 g), 9 g
• Chai-hu (Radix Bupleuri, 4 to 16 g), 9 g
• Dang-Gui (Radix Angelicae Sinensis, 5 to
11 g), 9 g • Fu-ling (Poria, 7 to 14 g),
15 g • Gan-cao (Radix Glycyrrhizae, 2 to
11 g), 6 g

194
Formula: Xiao-Zhi-Tang (3377)

消脂湯

Ingredients:
Fu-ling (Poria, 7 to 14 g), 15 g • He-ye
(Folium Nelumbinis, 4 to 11 g), 12 g •
Ju-hua (Flos Chrysanthemi, 4 to 20 g),
12 g • Jue-ming-zi (Semen Cassiae, 7 to
18 g), 15 g • Ren-dong-teng (Caulis
Lonicerae, 11 to 35 g), 15 g • Yi-yi-ren
(Semen Coicis, 11 to 22 g), 15 g • Yu-mi-
xu (Stigma Maydis, 30 to 60 g), 10 g •
Ze-xie (Rhizoma Alismatis, 7 to 14 g),
12 g

195
Formula: Xie-Gan-An-Shen-Wan (3372)

瀉肝安神丸

Ingredients:
Bai-zi-ren (Semen Biotae, 4 to 11 g), 10 g
• Che-qian-zi (Semen Plantaginis, 4 to
11 g), 10 g • Ci-ji-li (Fructus Tribuli, 7
to 10 g), 10 g • Dang-gui (Radix
Angelicae Sinensis, 5 to 11 g), 10 g • Fu-
shen (Buyury with pine root, 11 to 15 g),
10 g • Gan-cao (Radix Glycyrrhizae, 2 to
11 g), 3 g • Huang-qin (Radix
Scutellariae, 4 to 15 g), 10 g • Long-dan
(Radix Gentianae, 7 to 10 g), 10 g •
Long-gu (Os Draconis, 11 to 18 g), 10 g •
Mai-men-dong (Radix Ophiopogonis, 5 to
11 g), 10 g • Mu-li (Concha Ostrae, 11 to
35 g), 10 g • Sheng-di (Radix Rehmanniae,
14 to 35 g), 30 g • Shi-jue-ming (Concha
Haliotidis, 11 to 35 g), 30 g • Suan-zao-
ren (Semen Ziziphi Spinosae, 7 to 18 g),
10 g • Yuan-zhi (Radix Polygalae, 4 to
11 g), 10 g • Ze-xie (Rhizoma Alismatis, 7
to 14 g), 10 g • Zhen-zhu-mu (Concha

Margaritifera Usta, 10 to 30 g), 30 g •
Zhi-zi (Fructus Gardeniae, 7 to 16 g), 10 g

196
Formula: *Xie-Xin-Tang* (0367)

瀉心湯

Ingredients:
Da-haung (Radix Et Rhizoma Rhei, 4 to
15 g), 9 g • *Huang-lian (Rhizoma
Coptidis*, 2 to 12 g), 6 g • *Huang-qin
(Radix Scutellariae*, 4 to 15 g), 6 g

197
Formula: *Xin-Jia-Xiang-Ru-Yin* (0012 C)

新加香薷飲

Ingredients:
Bian-dou-hua (Flos Dolichoris, 5 to 11 g),
12 g • *Hou-po (Cortex Magnoliae
Officinalis*, 4 to 11 g), 9 g • *Jin-yin-hua
(Flos Lonicerae*, 7 to 18 g), 12 g • *Lian-
qiao (Fructus Forsythiae*, 5 to 11 g), 9 g •
Xiang-ru (Herba Elsholtziae Seu Moslae, 4
to 10 g), 9 g

198
Formula: *Xing-Su-San* (0046)

杏蘇散

Ingredients:
Ban-xia (Rhizoma Pinelliae, 4 to 12 g),
10 g • *Da-zao (Fructus Ziziphi Jujubae*, 7
to 18 g), three dates • *Fu-ling (Poria*, 7
to 14 g), 12 g • *Gan-cao (Radix
Glycyrrhizae*, 2 to 11 g), 2 g • *Jie-geng
(Radix Platycodi*, 2 to 5 g), 6 g • *Ju-pi
(Tangerine peel*, 3 to 17 g), 6 g • *Qian-
hu (Radix Peucedani*, 5 to 11 g), 6 g •
Sheng-jiang (Rhizoma Zingiberis Recens, 4
to 10 g), 6 g • *Xing-ren (Semen
Armeniacae Amarae*, 5 to 11 g), 9 g •
Zhi-qiao (Fructus Aurantii, 4 to 11 g), 6 g
• *Zi-su-ye (Folium Perillae*, 5 to 10 g), 6 g

199
Formula: *Xuan-Fu-Dai-Zhe-Tang* (0096)

旋復代赭湯

Ingredients:
Ban-xia (Rhizoma Pinelliae, 4 to 12 g),
12 g • *Da-zao (Fructus Ziziphi Jujubae*, 7
to 18 g), four dates • *Dai-zhe-shi
(Ocherum Rubrum*, 1 to 35 g), 30 g •
Gan-cao (Radix Glycyrrhizae, 2 to 11 g),
6 g • *Ren-shen (Radix Ginseng*, 1 to 35 g),
9 g • *Sheng-jiang (Rhizoma Zingiberis
Recens*, 4 to 10 g), 9 g • *Xuan-fu-hua
(Flos Inulae*, 4 to 11 g), 15 g

200
Formula: *Xue-Fu-Zhu-Yu-Tang* (0198)

血府逐瘀湯

Ingredients:
Chai-hu (Radix Bupleuri, 4 to 16 g), 9 g •
Chi-shao-yao (Radix Paeoniae Rubra, 5 to
11 g), 9 g • *Chuan-xiong (Rhizoma
Ligustici Chuanxiong*, 2 to 6 g), 6 g •
Dang-gui (Radix Angelicae Sinensis, 5 to
11 g), 12 g • *Gan-cao (Radix
Glycyrrhizae*, 2 to 11 g), 3 g • *Hong-hua
(Flos Carthami*, 4 to 7 g), 9 g • *Jie-geng
(Radix Platycodi*, 2 to 5 g), 6 g • *Niu-xi
(Radix Achyranthis Bidentatae*, 5 to 11 g),
12 g • *Sheng-di (Radix Rehmanniae*, 14 to
35 g), 12 g • *Tao-ren (Semen Persicae*, 5
to 11 g), 9 g • *Zhi-qiao (Fructus Aurantii*,
4 to 11 g), 9 g

201
Formula: *Yang-Jing-Zhong-Yu-Tang* (0652)

養精種玉湯

Ingredients:
Bai-shao-yao (Radix Paeoniae Alba, 5 to
11 g), 15 g • *Dang-gui (Radix Angelicae
Sinensis*, 5 to 11 g), 15 g • *Shan-zhu-yu
(Fructus Corni*, 5 to 11 g), 15 g • *Shu-di-
huang (Radix Rehmanniae Praeparatae*, 11
to 18 g), 15 g

202
Formula: *Yang-Xin-Tang* (1212)

養心湯

Ingredients:

Bai-zi-ren (Semen Biotae, 4 to 11 g), 8 g • Ban-xia-qu (Pinelliae mixture, 7 to 10 g), 15 g • *Chuan-xiong (Rhizoma Ligustici Chuanxiong 2 to 6 g), 15 g • Dang-gui (Radix Angelicae Sinensis, 5 to 11 g), 15 g • Fu-ling (Poria, 7 to 14 g), 15 g • Fu-shen (Buyury* with pine root, 11 to 15 g), 15 g • *Gan-cao (Radix Glycyrrhizae, 2 to 11 g), 12 g • Huang-qi (Radix Astragali Seu Hedysari, 5 to 40 g), 15 g • Ren-shen (Radix Ginseng, 1 to 35 g), 8 g • Rou-gui (Cortex Cinnamomi, 1 to 5 g), 8 g • Suan-zao-ren (Semen Ziziphi Spinosae, 7 to 18 g), 8 g • Wu-wei-zi (Fructus Schisandrae, 2 to 4 g), 8 g • Yuan-zhi (Radix Polygalae, 4 to 11 g), 8 g*

203
Formula: *Yang-Yin-Qing-Fei-Tang (0050)*

養陰清肺湯

Ingredients:

Bai-shao-yao (Radix Paeoniae Alba, 5 to 11 g), 12 g • Bo-he (Herba Menthae, 3 to 10 g), 6 g • Chuan-bei-mu (Bulbus Fritillariae Cirrhosae, 4 to 14 g), 10 g • Gan-cao (Radix Glycyrrhizae, 2 to 11 g), 6 g • Mai-men-dong (Radix Ophiopogonis, 5 to 11 g), 20 g • Mu-dan-pi (Cortex Moutan Radicis, 5 to 11 g), 12 g • Sheng-di (Radix Rehmanniae, 14 to 35 g), 30 g • Xuan-shen (Radix Scrophulariae, 7 to 35 g), 24 g

204
Formula: *Yang-Yin-Tong-Bi-Tang (2930)*

養陰通痹湯

Ingredients:

Dang-shen (Radix Codonopsis Pilosulae, 11 to 15 g), 12 g • Gua-lou (Fructus Trichosanthis, 11 to 15 g), 18 g • Hong-hua (Flos Carthami, 4 to 7 g), 6 g • Mai-men-dong (Radix Ophiopogonis, 5 to 11 g), 12 g • Nu-zhen-zi (Fructus Ligustri Lucidi, 5 to 11 g), 15 g • Sheng-di (Radix Rehmanniae, 14 to 35 g), 18 g • Tao-ren (Semen Persicae, 5 to 11 g), 10 g • Wu-wei-zi (Fructus Schisandrae, 2 to 4 g), 10 g • Yan-hu-suo (Rhizoma Corydalis, 4 to 11 g), 10 g

205
Formula: *Yi-Gong-San (0533)*

异功散

Ingredients:

Bai-zhu (Rhizoma Atractylodis Macrocephalae, 5 to 11 g), 10 g • Chen-pi (Pericarpium Citri Reticulatae Viride, 4 to 11 g), 10 g • Fu-ling (Poria, 7 to 14 g), 12 g • Gan-cao (Radix Glycyrrhizae, 2 to 11 g), 3 g • Ren-shen (Radix Ginseng, 1 to 35 g), 15 g

206
Formula: *Yi-Guan-Jian (0240)*

一貫煎

Ingredients:

Chuan-lian-zi (Fructus Meliae Toosendan, 5 to 11 g), 6 g • Dang-gui (Radix Angelicae Sinensis, 5 to 11 g), 9 g • Gou-qi-zi (Fructus Lycii, 5 to 11 g), 9 g • Mai-men-dong (Radix Ophiopogonis, 5 to 11 g), 9 g • Nan-sha-shen (Radix Adenophorae, 5 to 11 g), 9 g • Sheng-di (Radix Rehmanniae, 14 to 35 g), 18 g

207
Formula: *Yi-Wei-Tang (0136)*

益胃湯

Ingredients:

Bing-tang (Rock Sugar, flexible g), flexible quantity • Mai-men-dong (Radix Ophiopogonis, 5 to 11 g), 15 g • Nan-sha-shen (Radix Adenophorae, 5 to 11 g), 10 g • Sheng-di (Radix Rehmanniae, 14 to 35 g), 30 g • Yu-zhu (Rhizoma Polygonati Odorath, 5 to 11 g), 10 g

208
Formula: *Yi-Yi-Ren-Tang (1477)*

薏苡仁湯

Ingredients:
Cang-zhu (Rhizoma Atractylodis Macrocephalae, 4 to 11 g), 11 g • Cao-wu (Radix Aconiti/Radix Aconiti Kusnezoffii, 2 to 5 g), 5 g • Chuan-xiong (Rhizoma Ligustici Chuanxiong, 2 to 6 g), 6 g • Dang-gui (Radix Angelicae Sinensis, 5 to 11 g), 11 g • Du-huo (Radix Angelicae Pubescentis, 2 to 5 g), 5 g • Fang-feng (Radix Ledebouriellae, 5 to 10 g), 10 g • Gan-cao (Radix Glycyrrhizae, 2 to 11 g), 11 g • Gui-zhi (Ramulus Cinnamomi, 2 to 10 g), 10 g • Ma-huang (Herba Ephedrae, 5 to 10 g), 10 g • Qiang-huo (Rhizoma Seu Radix Notopterygii, 4 to 10 g), 10 g • Sheng-jiang (Rhizoma Zingiberis Recens, 4 to 10 g), 10 g • Yi-yi-ren (Semen Coicis, 11 to 22 g), 22 g
Instructions: Grind into powder, and take 6 g of powder twice daily.

209
Formula: Yin-Chen-Hao-Tang (0261)

茵陳蒿湯

Ingredients:
Da-huang (Radix Et Rhizoma Rhei, 4 to 15 g), 9 g • Yin-chen (Herba Artemisiae Scopariae, 7 to 21 g), 60 g • Zhi-zi (Fructus Gardeniae, 7 to 16 g), 9 g

210
Formula: Yin-Chen-Wu-Ling-San (0348B)

茵陳五苓散

Ingredients:
Bai-zhu (Rhizoma Atractylodis Macrocephalae, 5 to 11 g), 9 g • Fu-ling (Poria, 7 to 14 g), 12 g • Gui-zhi (Ramulus Cinnamomi, 2 to 10 g), 9 g • Yin-chen-hao (Herba Artemisiae Capillaris, 10 to 18 g), 9 g • Ze-xie (Rhizoma Alismatis, 7 to 14 g), 15 g • Zhu-ling (Polyporus Umbellatus, 7 to 14 g), 12 g

211
Formula: Yin-Chen-Zhu-Fu-Tang (0656)

茵陳术附湯

Ingredients:
Bai-zhu (Rhizoma Atractylodis Macrocephalae, 5 to 11 g), 6 g • Fu-zi (Radix Aconiti Praeparata, 4 to 11 g), 2 g • Gan-cao (Radix Glycyrrhizae, 2 to 11 g), 3 g • Gan-jiang (Rhizoma Zingiberis, 3 to 7 g), 2 g • Rou-gui (Cortex Cinnamomi, 1 to 5 g), 1 g • Yin-chen (Herba Artemisiae Capillaris/Herba Artemisiae Scopariae Scopariae, 7 to 21 g), 3 g

212
Formula: Yin-Qiao-San (0015)

銀翹散

Ingredients:
Bo-he (Herba Menthae, 3 to 10 g), 18 g • Dou-chi (Semen Sojae Praeparatum, 10 to 15 g), 15 g • Gan-cao (Radix Glycyrrhizae, 2 to 11 g), 9 g • Jie-geng (Radix Platycodi, 2 to 5 g), 6 g • Jin-yin-hua (Flos Lonicerae, 7 to 18 g), 30 g • Jing-jie (Herba Schizonepetae, 5 to 10 g), 18 g • Lian-qiao (Fructus Forsythiae, 5 to 11 g), 30 g • Lu-gen (Rhizoma Phragmitis, 15 to 65 g), 30 g • Niu-bang-zi (Fructus Arctii, 6 to 10 g), 18 g • Zhu-ye (Folium Bambusae, 4 to 20 g), 12 g

213
Formula: You-Gui-Wan (0963)

右歸丸

Ingredients:
Dang-gui (Radix Angelicae Sinensis, 5 to 11 g), 90 g • Du-zhong (Cortex Eucommiae, 7 to 11 g), 120 g • Fu-zi (Radix Aconiti Praeparata, 4 to 11 g), 60 g • Gou-qi-zi (Fructus Lych, 5 to 11 g), 120 g • Lu-jiao-jiao (Colla Cornus Cervi, X g), 120 g • Rou-gui (Cortex Cinnamomi, 1 to 5 g), 60 g • Shan-yao (Rhizoma Dioscoreae Bulbiferae, 10 to 20 g), 120 g • Shan-zhu-yu (Fructus Corni, 5 to 11 g), 90 g • Shu-di-huang (Radix Rehmanniae Praeparatae, 11 to 18 g), 240 g • Tu-si-zi (Semen Cuscutae, 5 to 11 g), 120 g

Instructions: Grind into powder to make tablets, and take 15 g of tablets twice daily.

214
Formula: *You-Gui-Yin* (0331D)

右歸飲

Ingredients:
Du-zhong (Cortex Eucommiae, 7 to 11 g), 120 g • *Fu-zi (Radix Aconiti Praeparata, 4 to 11 g)*, 30 g • *Gan-cao (Radix Glycyrrhizae, 2 to 11 g)*, 15 g • *Gan-di (Dried Radix Rehmanniae, 11 to 18 g)*, 240 g • *Gou-qi-zi (Fructus Lych, 5 to 11 g)*, 120 g • *Rou-gui (Cortex Cinnamomi, 1 to 5 g)*, 30 g • *Shan-yao (Rhizoma Dioscoreae, 10 to 20 g)*, 120 g • *Shan-zhu-yu (Fructus Corni, 5 to 11 g)*, 120 g

Instructions: Grind into powder to make tablets with honey. Take 9 g of tablets one to two times daily, with warm or lightly salted water. Use reduced quantities of ingredients if decoction is done.

215
Formula: *Yu-Nu-Jian* (0476)

玉女煎

Ingredients:
Mai-men-dong (Radix Ophiopogonis, 5 to 11 g), 6 g • *Nu-xi (Radix Achyranthis Bidentatae, 5 to 11 g)*, 5 g • *Shi-gao (Gypsum Fibrosum, 10 to 70 g)*, 30 g • *Shu-di-huang (Radix Rehmanniae Praeparatae, 11 to 18 g)*, 15 g • *Zhi-mu (Rhizoma Anemarrhenae, 4 to 15 g)*, 5 g

216
Formula: *Yu-Ping-Feng-San* (0022)

玉屏風散

Ingredients:
Bai-zhu (Rhizoma Atractylodis Macrocephalae, 5 to 11 g), 9 g • *Fang-feng (Radix Ledebouriellae, 5 to 10 g)*, 9 g • *Huang-qi (Radix Astragali Seu Hedysari, 5 to 40 g)*, 24 g

217
Formula: *Yue-Bi-Jia-Zhu-Tang* (0053)

越婢加朮湯

Ingredients:
Bai-zhu (Rhizoma Atractylodis Macrocephalae, 5 to 11 g), 10 g • *Da-zao (Fructus Ziziphi Jujubae, 7 to 18 g)*, 12 g • *Gan-cao (Radix Glycyrrhizae, 2 to 11 g)*, 3 g • *Ma-huang (Herba Ephedrae, 5 to 10 g)*, 10 g • *Sheng-jiang (Rhizoma Zingiberis Recens, 4 to 10 g)*, 10 g • *Shi-gao (Gypsum Fibrosum, 10 to 70 g)*, 40 g

218
Formula: *Yue-Bi-Tang* (0051)

越婢湯

Ingredients:
Da-zao (Fructus Ziziphi Jujubae, 7 to 18 g), 10 g • *Gan-cao (Radix Glycyrrhizae, 2 to 11 g)*, 6 g • *Ma-huang (Herba Ephedrae, 5 to 10 g)*, 15 g • *Sheng-jiang (Rhizoma Zingiberis Recens, 4 to 10 g)*, 9 g • *Shi-gao (Gypsum Fibrosum, 10 to 70 g)*, 50 g

219
Formula: *Yue-Hua-Wan* (0468)

月華丸

Ingredients:
Bai-bu (Radix Stemonae, 4 to 7 g), 60 g • *Bei-sha-shen (Radix Glehniae, 5 to 11 g)*, 60 g • *Chuan-bei-mu (Bulbus Fritillariae Thunbergii Cirrhosae, 4 to 14 g)*, 21 g • *E-jiao (Colla Corii Asini, 5 to 11 g)*, 21 g • *Fu-ling (Poria, 7 to 14 g)*, 60 g • *Ju-hua (Flos Chrysanthemi, 4 to 20 g)*, 60 g • *Mai-men-dong (Radix Ophiopogonis, 5 to 11 g)*, 30 g • *San-qi (Radix Notoginseng, 2 to 10 g)*, 15 g • *Sang-ye (Folium Mori, 5 to 10 g)*, 60 g • *Shan-yao (Rhizoma*

Dioscoreae, 10 to 20 g), 60 g • *Sheng-di (Radix Rehmanniae, 14 to 35 g), 60 g • Shu-di-huang (Radix Rehmanniae Praeparatae, 11 to 18 g), 60 g • Tian-Dong (Radix Asparagi, 7 to 14 g), 30 g*
Instructions: Grind into powder, and take 9 g of powder twice daily.

220
Formula: *Zeng-Yi-Cheng-Qi-Tang* (0155)
增液承氣湯

Ingredients:
Da-huang (Radix Et Rhizoma Rhei, 4 to 15 g), 6 g • Mai-men-dong (Radix Ophiopogonis, 5 to 11 g), 12 g • Pu-xiao Mirabilitum Depuratum, 5 to 11 g), 5 g • Sheng-di (Radix Rehmanniae, 14 to 35 g), 24 g • Xuan-shen (Radix Scrophulariae, 7 to 35 g), 24 g

221
Formula: *Zeng-Yi-Tang* (0138)
增液湯

Ingredients:
Mai-men-dong (Radix Ophiopogonis, 5 to 11 g), 24 g • Sheng-di (Radix Rehmanniae (fresh), 14 to 35 g), 24 g • Xuan-shen (Radix Scrophulariae, 7 to 35 g), 30 g

222
Formula: *Zhen-Gan-Xi-Feng-Tang* (0242)
鎮肝熄風湯

Ingredients:
Bai-shao-yao (Radix Paeoniae Alba, 5 to 11 g), 15 g • Chuan-lian-zi (Fructus Meliae Toosendan, 5 to 11 g), 6 g • Dai-zhe-shi (Ocherum Rubrum, 1 to 35 g), 15 g • Gan-cao (Radix Glycyrrhizae, 2 to 11 g), 4 g • Gui-ban (Plastrum Testudinis, 11 to 30 g), 15 g • Long-gu (Os Draconis, 11 to 18 g), 15 g • Mai-ya (Fructus Hordei Germinatus, 11 to 13 g), 6 g • Mu-li (Concha Ostrae, 11 to 35 g), 15 g • Niu-xi (Radix Achyranthis Bidentatae, 5 to

11 g), 30 g • *Tian-dong (Radix Asparagi, 7 to 14 g), 15 g • Xuan-shen (Radix Scrophulariae, 7 to 35 g), 15 g • Yin-chen (Herba Artemisiae Scopariae, 7 to 21 g), 15 g*

223
Formula: *Zhen-Wu-Tang* (0347)
真武湯

Ingredients:
Bai-zhu (Rhizoma Atractylodis Macrocephalae, 5 to 11 g), 9 to 15 g • Chi-Shao-yao (Radix Paeoniae Rubra, 5 to 11 g), 9 to 18 g • Fu-ling (Poria, 7 to 14 g), 15 to 24 g • Fu-zi (Radix Aconiti Praeparata, 4 to 11 g), 15 to 60 g • Sheng-jiang (Rhizoma Zingiberis Recens, 4 to 10 g), 9 to 18 g
Instructions: Decoct fu-zi over low heat for half an hour, add the remaining ingredients to the decoction, and divide into three doses for one-day consumption; drink it warm.

224
Formula: *Zhi-Bai-Di-Huang-Wan* (0327E)
知柏地黃丸

Ingredients:
Fu-ling (Poria, 7 to 14 g), 90 g • Huang-bai (Cortex Phellodendri, 4 to 15 g), 90 g • Mu-dan-pi (Cortex Moutan Radicis, 5 to 11 g), 90 g • Shan-yao (Rhizoma Dioscoreae, 10 to 20 g), 120 g • Shan-zhu-yu (Fructus Corni, 5 to 11 g), 120 g • Shu-di-huang (Radix Rehmanniae Praeparatae, 11 to 18 g), 240 g • Ze-xie (Rhizoma Alismatis, 7 to 14 g), 90 g • Zhi-mu (Rhizoma Anemarrhenae, 4 to 15 g), 90 g
Instructions: Grind into powder to make tablets, and take three tablets or 9 g two to three times daily.

225
Formula: *Zhi-Bao-Dan* (0288)
至寶丹

Ingredients:

An-xi-xiang (Benzoinum, 0.3 to 2 g), 45 g • Bing-pian (Borneol, 0.2 to 0.3 g), 3 g • Dai-mao (Carapax Eretmochelydis, 4 to 7 g), 30 g • Hu-po (Succinum, 1 to 2 g), 30 g • Niu-huang (Calculus bovis, 0.2 to 0.5 g), 15 g • She-xiang (Moschus, 0.01 to 0.03 g), 3 g • Xi-jiao (Cornu Rhinoceri, 1 to 2 g), 30 g • Xiong-huang (Realgar, 0.3 to 1.5 g), 30 g • Zhu-sha (Cinnabaris, 0.3 to 1 g), 30 g

Instructions: Grind into powder to make tablets, and take one tablet or 3 g each time. (Patent medicine also available.)

226
Formula: *Zhi-Gan-Cao-Tang* (0311)

炙甘草湯

Ingredients:

Da-zao (Fructus Ziziphi Jujubae, 7 to 18 g), 12 g • E-jiao (Colla Corii Asini, 5 to 11 g), 12 g • Gan-cao, zhi-gan-cao (Radix Glycyrrhizae, 2 to 11 g), 15 g • Gui-zhi (Ramulus Cinnamomi, 2 to 10 g), 9 g • Huo-ma-ren (Fructus Cannabis, 11 to 17 g), 15 g • Mai-men-dong (Radix Ophiopogonis, 5 to 11 g), 9 g • Ren-shen (Radix Ginseng, 1 to 35 g), 9 g • Sheng-jiang (Rhizoma Zingiberis Recens, 4 to 10 g), 9 g • Shu-di-huang (Radix Rehmanniae Praeparatae, 11 to 18 g), 30 g

227
Formula: *Zhi-Shi-Dao-Zhi-Wan* (0075)

枳實導滯丸

Ingredients:

Bai-zhu (Rhizoma Atractylodis Macrocephalae, 5 to 11 g), 10 g • Da-Huang (Radix Et Rhizoma Rhei, 4 to 15 g), 10 g • Fu-ling (Poria, 7 to 14 g), 10 g • Huang-lian (Rhizoma Coptidis, 2 to 12 g), 10 g • Huang-qin (Radix Scutellariae, 4 to 15 g), 10 g • Shen-qu (Massa Medicata Fermentata, 7 to 15 g), 12 g • Ze-xie (Rhizoma Alismatis, 7 to 14 g), 6 g • Zhi-shi (Fructus Aurantii Immaturus, 4 to 7 g), 10 g

228 • **Formula**: *Zhi-Shi-Xie-Bai-Gui-Zhi-Tang* (0215C)

枳實薤白桂枝湯

Ingredients:

Gua-lou (Fructus Trichosanthis, 11 to 15 g), 24 g • Gui-zhi (Ramulus Cinnamomi, 2 to 10 g), 10 g • Hou-po (Cortex Magnoliae Officinalis, 4 to 11 g), 12 g • Xie-bai (Bulbus Allii Macrostemi, 5 to 11 g), 30 g • Zhi-shi (Fructus Aurantii Immaturus, 4 to 7 g), 12 g

229
Formula: *Zhu-Ye-Shi-Gao-Tang* (0545)

竹葉石膏湯

Ingredients:

Ban-xia (Rhizoma Pinelliae, 4 to 12 g), 12 g • Gan-cao (Radix Glycyrrhizae, 2 to 11 g), 6 g • Jing-mi (polished rice, flexible quantity), 10 g • Mai-men-dong (Radix Ophiopogonis, 5 to 11 g) 30 g • Ren-shen (Radix Ginseng, 1 to 35 g), 6 g • Shi-gao (Gypsum Fibrosum, 10 to 70 g), 30 g • Zhu-ye (Folium Bambusae, 4 to 20 g), 10 g

230
Formula: *Zi-Shen-Yang-Xue-Jian-Bu-Tang* (3378)

滋腎養血健步湯

Ingredients:

Bai-shao-yao (Radix Paeoniae Alba, 5 to 11 g), 12 g • Dang-gui (Radix Angelicae Sinensis, 5 to 11 g), 12 g • Du-zhong (Cortex Eucommiae, 7 to 11 g), 12 g • Gou-qi-zi (Fructus Lycii, 5 to 11 g), 12 g • Gou-teng (Ramulus Uncariae Cum Uncis, 5 to 11 g), 30 g • Gui-ban (Plastrum Testudinis, 11 to 30 g), 30 g • Huang-qi (Radix Astragali Seu Hedysari, 5 to 40 g), 30 g • Jiang-can (Bombyx Batryticatus, 5 to 11 g), 15 g • Niu-xi (Radix Achyranthis Bidentatae, 5 to 11 g), 15 g • Rou-gui (Cortex Cinnamomi, 1 to 5 g), 6 g

• Sha-wan-zi (Semen Astragalus, 7 to 11 g), 12 g • Shu-di-huang (Radix Rehmanniae Praeparatae, 11 to 18 g), 30 g • Tu-si-zi (Semen Cuscutae, 5 to 11 g), 12 g

231
Formula: Zuo-Gui-Wan (0962)

左歸丸

Ingredients:
Gou-qi-zi (Fructus Lycii, 5 to 11 g), 120 g • Gui-ban-jiao (Colla Plastri Testudinis, 3 to 10 g), 120 g • Lu-jiao-jiao (Colla cornus Cervi, 6 to 12 g), 120 g • Niu-xi (Radix Achyranthis Bidentatae, 5 to 11 g), 90 g • Shan-yao (Rhizoma Dioscoreae Bulbiferae, 10 to 20 g), 120 g • Shan-zhu-yu (Fructus Corni, 5 to 11 g), 120 g • Shu-di-huang (Radix Rehmanniae

Praeparatae, 11 to 18 g), 240 g • Tu-si-zi (Semen Cuscutae, 5 to 11 g), 120 g

Instructions: Grind into powder to make tablets, and take 9 g of tablets twice daily.

232
Formula: Zuo-Gui-Yin (0328)

左歸飲

Ingredients:
Fu-ling (Poria, 7 to 14 g), 6 g • Gan-cao, zhi-gan-cao (Radix Glycyrrhizae, 2 to 11 g), 3 g • Gou-qi-zi (Fructus Lycii, 5 to 11 g), 6 g • Shan-yao (Rhizoma Dioscoreae, 10 to 20 g), 6 g • Shan-zhu-yu (Fructus Corni, 5 to 11 g), 3 to 6 g (reduce in case of fear of cold) • Shu-di-huang (Radix Rehmanniae Praeparatae, 11 to 18 g), 6 to 10 g (or as much as 30 to 60 g)

GUIDE TO APPROXIMATE EQUIVALENTS

CUSTOMARY				METRIC
Ounces Pounds	Cups	Tablespoons	Teaspoons	Grams Kilograms
			¼ t.	1.25 g
			½ t.	2.5 g
			1 t.	5 g
			2 t.	10 g
½ oz.		1 T.	3 t.	15 g
1 oz.		2 T.	6 t.	30 g
2 oz.	¼ c.	4 T.	12 t.	60 g
4 oz.	½ c.	8 T.	24 t.	120 g
8 oz.	1 c.	16 T.	48 t.	240 g
1 lb.	2 c.			480 g
2 lb.	4 c.			
2.2 lb.				1 kg

Keep in mind that this is not an exact conversion, but generally may be used in measuring herbs.

INDEX